Critical Hospital Social

Critical Hospital Social Work Practice sheds light on the fast-paced, high pressure role of the hospital social worker. At a time of public concern over the state of the NHS and the needs of a growing older population, the hospital social worker's job is more important than ever. Yet, it is poorly understood and often overlooked by policy makers, managers and other professionals.

Employing social theory to make sense of the contemporary context of health and social care, this book highlights the vital role played by social workers in planning complex hospital discharges. It provides an in-depth account of the activities of a typical hospital social work team in the UK, drawn from rigorous ethnographic fieldwork, and contrasts this with research evidence on hospital social work practices around the world. The author points towards exciting new directions for health-related social work and social work's potential to develop critical gerontological practice.

This book will be useful to social work students and practitioners working in hospital settings and with older people in general. It will also be of significant value to policy makers and academics who are interested in developing innovative approaches to meeting the needs of the ageing population.

Daniel Burrows trained as a social worker at Cardiff University, where he and his future wife met. After seven years in practice, he moved over to teaching and completed his professional doctorate. He now lives in Cardiff with his wife and two sons and teaches on the MA Social Work at Cardiff University.

Routledge Advances in Social Work

Conversation Analysis for Social Work
Talking with Youth in Care
Gerald deMontigny

Older Lesbian, Gay, Bisexual and Trans People
Minding the Knowledge Gap
Andrew King, Kathryn Almack, Yiu-Tung Suen and Sue Westwood

Visual Communication for Social Work Practice
Power, Culture, Analysis
Sonia Magdalena Tascon

Art in Social Work Practice
Theory and Practice: International Perspectives
Ephrat Huss and Eltje Bos

The Uses and Abuses of Humour in Social Work
Stephen Jordan

Eco-Social Transformation and Community-Based Economy
Susanne Elsen

The International Development of Social Work Education
The Vietnam Experience
Edward Cohen, Alice Hines, Laurie Drabble, Hoa Nguyen, Meekung Han, Soma Sen and Debra Faires

International Perspectives on Social Work and Political Conflict
Edited by Joe Duffy, Jim Campbell and Carol Tosone

Asian Social Work
Professional Work in National Contexts
Edited by Ian Shaw and Rosaleen Ow

Critical Hospital Social Work Practice
Daniel Burrows

For more information about this series, please visit: https://www.routledge.com/Routledge-Advances-in-Social-Work/book-series/RASW

Critical Hospital Social Work Practice

Daniel Burrows

Routledge
Taylor & Francis Group

LONDON AND NEW YORK

First published 2020 by Routledge

2 Park Square, Milton Park, Abingdon, Oxon OX14 4RN

605 Third Avenue, New York, NY 10017

Routledge is an imprint of the Taylor & Francis Group, an informa business

First issued in paperback 2022

British Library Cataloguing-in-Publication Data
A catalogue record for this book is available from the British Library

Library of Congress Cataloging-in-Publication Data
Names: Burrows, Daniel, author.
Title: Critical hospital social work practice / Daniel Burrows.
Description: Milton Park, Abingdon, Oxon ; New York,
NY : Routledge, 2020. |
Series: Routledge advances in social work | Includes bibliographical references and index.
Identifiers: LCCN 2019058405 (print) | LCCN 2019058406 (ebook) |
ISBN 9780367203849 (hardback) | ISBN 9780429261213 (ebook)
Subjects: LCSH: Medical social work--England.
Classification: LCC HV687.5.G7 B87 2020 (print) |
LCC HV687.5.G7 (ebook) | DDC 362.1/0425--dc23
LC record available at https://lccn.loc.gov/2019058405
LC ebook record available at https://lccn.loc.gov/2019058406

ISBN: 978-0-367-20384-9 (hbk)
ISBN: 978-1-03-233637-4 (pbk)
DOI: 10.4324/9780429261213

Typeset in Times New Roman
by Taylor & Francis Books

Dedicated to the memory of
Clive Burrows 22 January 1946 – 5 February 2000
and
Roger Alexander 27 December 1948 – 15 October 2019

Contents

Acknowledgements   viii

PART I
Key issues in hospital social work   1

1   Hospital social work in context   3

2   A brief history of hospital social work   19

3   The current state of hospital social work   34

4   Using research in social work   47

PART II
An ethnographic account of hospital social work   61

5   Social work in the 'iron cage'   63

6   Is it still social work?   79

7   The social work 'cuckoo' in the hospital 'nest'   97

8   Conclusions   115

    References   128
    Index   146

Acknowledgements

I am deeply grateful to the hospital social workers who were generous enough to allow me into their world and were so welcoming and friendly. When I finished the fieldwork, I left with deep admiration of their commitment to the well-being of the patients and carers with whom they work. My gratitude also extends to the clinicians and nurse managers who participated in my research with such friendliness and willingness, and to the patients and carers who did likewise.

I am much indebted to my two doctoral supervisors, Teresa de Villiers and Jonathan Scourfield, for their guidance and support. I must express my thanks to my wife, Hannah, for all the many ways she has supported me in this work and to our two boys, Frank and Wilfred, who have been an inspiration since their arrival, as well as a welcome antidote to the hard graft of academia. I am grateful for the support and encouragement of colleagues at Cardiff Met and Cardiff University and also wish to thank Geoff Underwood, Kris Ellis and David Mellor for the joy of their friendship. Finally, I must thank my mother, Diane Burrows, who has always supported me in pursuing my goals.

Part I

Key issues in hospital social work

Preface

This book is concerned with statutory social work as it is practised by teams of hospital-based social workers employed by local authorities in hospitals all over the UK. Typically, these teams work almost exclusively with older people who are inpatients and who are unable to be discharged safely without social work services because of social care needs that have come to light since their admission. Hospital social workers are responsible for arranging services for such patients to be discharged as quickly as possible. This involves making an assessment of the patient's needs, taking into account the views of the patient, clinicians and family members/carers, and producing a plan of services to enable the patient to be discharged safely from hospital. Typically, the care plan will arrange either for care services to come to the patient's home or for the patient to go into residential care. The social care needs of patients usually arise from declining physical health, increasing physical disability and/or problems of cognition often related to dementia. Hospital social work is therefore characterised by short-term involvement with patients, whose cases are usually then passed on for review by community-based teams, and pressure from clinicians and hospital managers to deliver patient discharges as quickly as possible.

While I am concentrating exclusively on the mainstream statutory form of hospital social work, I fully acknowledge that there are other forms of social work that are practised by social workers based in hospitals around the UK. For example, as a practitioner, I spent six years working on a paediatric oncology unit, in a charitably funded post with the purpose of providing practical and emotional support for families while their children went through cancer treatment. While this niche role, and others similar to it, are of great merit and interest, they are so distinctive from the mainstream form of hospital social work as to be beyond the scope of this book.

Part I sets out the contemporary context of hospital social work and explores its historic development and current state, drawing comparisons with practices in other parts of the world. Part II explores an in-depth ethnographic study of a UK hospital social work team.

1 Hospital social work in context

Introduction

Since its foundation, health care has been the domain of the NHS, while responsibility for the provision of social care has resided with local authorities. Hospital social workers, who are usually employed by local authorities, therefore play a vital role in providing an interface between the health service and social provision, through discharge planning for those individuals who are in need of ongoing support in order to leave hospital (Moriarty et al., 2019). Primarily, hospital social work teams are occupied with discharge planning for elderly people whose medical and social needs are complex. This chapter examines the care of older people in hospitals, before going on to discuss social work with older people in the more broad sense, drawing especially on Bauman's concept of 'liquid modernity' (Bauman, 2000a; Bauman, 2007) to explore the contemporary social context of ageing within which social work practice occurs.

The ageing population and the NHS

> No society can legitimately call itself civilised if a sick person is denied medical aid because of a lack of means.
>
> (Bevan, 1952, p. 100)

The UK's National Health Service, established at the end of the Second World War, represents a bold and ambitious attempt by a state to provide a service to meet the needs and desires of all its citizens (Lowe, 2004). The vision of its founding secretary of state, Aneurin Bevan, was that it should provide all appropriate and necessary health care to both rich and poor, based on need, rather than means. In other words, the NHS was not to be merely a safety net for those who were unable to afford to make their own private arrangements, but a means of providing the best health care possible as a universal citizenship right (Rivett, 1998). This vision of the NHS was widely popular at its inception and continues to hold sway in the popular consciousness in the present day. Although a market in private health care and insurance flourishes for a small proportion of the population,[1] most of the UK population continue to expect the NHS to meet all their health needs without charge at the point of delivery (apart from dentistry and optometry). While expectations of the universality of NHS provision have not changed, however, both the needs of the population and the scope of medicine have evolved so far as to be completely transformed in the period since the NHS was established. The effects of these transformations on the care of older people are of great significance and must be understood by social workers who need to work with hospital systems, whether as part of hospital discharge teams or in community teams with responsibility for hospital patients.[2]

When the NHS was founded, the practice of medicine was far less complex and less costly than today. Fewer diseases were treatable and fewer people lived into advanced old age, meaning that the treatment of the sick was a simpler (though less frequently successful) process (Porter, 1999). The developing ability of medicine to overcome disease, with the emergence of new sciences and vast improvements in surgical techniques, pharmacotherapies, diagnostics and technologies, and the efficient distribution of modern medicine to the people at large through the NHS, have supported developments in the demographic composition of the UK population that create a different range of needs to those which the NHS was founded to meet. Of particular consequence in this regard is the increase in the numbers of people living into old age and the increasing life expectancy of people at age 65.

Shortly after the introduction of the NHS, life expectancy at birth in England and Wales was around 66 years for men and 72 years for women. A steady increase in overall life expectancy followed over subsequent decades, such that by 2012, a new-born boy could expect to live 79 years, while a new-born girl's life expectancy had lengthened to almost 83 years (Office for National Statistics, 2015). In 1997, around one in six people were aged 65 years and over; by 2017 that figure had increased to one in five people, and it is projected to reach around one in four people by 2037 (Office for National Statistics, 2018). For the NHS, a significant consequence of the growth of the ageing population is the increase in people living into advanced old age (i.e. 80+ years of age). In 1950–1952, a person who lived to the age of 80 would have a further life expectancy of around five years; by 2012 this had increased to nearly ten. As people progress through old age their health needs tend to become more complex and they are more likely to depend on assistance and support from others to manage daily living. The increase in the population of people in advanced old age has therefore given rise to a need for systems of complex health and social care provision, involving skilled and specialised clinicians[3] with expertise specific to the multiple and various challenges of ageing.

It is ironic that the success of medicine in improving longevity is born of professional and institutional systems that are ill-equipped to look after the ageing population that they have helped to create. The nature of medicine as both a practice and an academic discipline rests on its continuing refinement and improvement (Porter, 1999), meaning that doctors keep up a career-long pursuit of both extending their own personal knowledge and of contributing to the generation of new knowledge in the field. Hospitals have become not only centres in which to treat the sick, but also hubs in which the boundaries of scientific knowledge are extended through experimentation and improvisation. Doctors tend to specialise, and their knowledge and interests become deeper yet narrower as they rise in seniority. While this drive for advancing knowledge should be celebrated for improving the treatments available for patients' diseases, it must also be acknowledged that it creates a working climate in which both the self-esteem and prestige of doctors rests on the privileging of clinical, curative tasks over other forms of care that may be of equal or even greater importance to the patient (Latimer, 2000). As a result, elderly patients with complex co-morbidities become less attractive patients to treat, because a doctor's ability to treat one disease successfully does not necessarily result in the restoration of health to the patient.

Hospital care, of course, does not depend on doctors alone. The majority of the direct care of patients is carried out by nurses and health care assistants (and, of course, the contribution of a range of allied health care professionals including physiotherapists, occupational therapists, speech therapists etc. should not be overlooked). Just as medicine has been transformed by the continuing pursuit and development of applied scientific knowledge, nursing has undergone a similar revolution through the project of professionalisation (Yam, 2004; Gunn et al., 2019). Professionalisation has led to nurses taking on additional responsibilities that formerly would have been the preserve of physicians alone, including the administration and prescription of medication, collection and recording of diagnostic information and the diagnosis and treatment of minor injuries and conditions (Westbrook et al., 2011). All of these tasks result in an increased administrative burden on nurses both for the recording and co-ordination of treatments. As a result, qualified nurses have less time to spend in direct contact with patients and vital aspects of patient care are held in lower esteem and are left to less qualified workers (Gillen and Graffin, 2010). This is particularly problematic for older patients when suffering from dementia or confusion. Caring for people in a confused state requires considerable skill underpinned by theoretical knowledge, yet this crucial relational work is not easily recognised or accounted for and standards of nursing practice in this regard are variable (Dewing and Dijk, 2016).

The effect of both the ongoing development of medicine and the professionalisation of nursing is that wards and clinics have become spaces in which the emphasis is upon *cure* rather than *care*. This occupational and institutional culture can create difficulties for older people, since their medical presentations are often resistant to the linear trajectory of cure, due to the complexity of co-morbidities so frequently present in the ageing body. Older patients may find that their illnesses fall among a range of medical specialities, leaving the rightful location of their treatment within the hospital disputed (Tadd et al., 2011). In summary, because it is often so difficult to cure older people's diseases, responsibility for the care of individual older people within hospitals can be shunned instead of embraced both by individual practitioners and whole specialist teams or wards.

In addition to the unattractiveness to clinicians of treating older people whose bodies are resistant to straightforward cure, the development of risk management practices within contemporary health care has resulted in the prioritisation of a rational response to patients' bodily needs over holistic approaches that incorporate emotional and psychological needs (Hillman et al., 2013). For example, as a response to the risk of elderly patients having falls, ward staff sometimes encourage continent individuals to soil pads rather than help them to the toilet, and the risk of the spread of infection results in patients being left isolated in side rooms (Calnan et al., 2013). Such measures make sense in terms of risk management, but can be detrimental to older people's sense of dignity and emotional well-being. These issues do not arise in the main because hospital staff set out deliberately to treat older people badly (though abuse by professionals of all backgrounds must be guarded against), but the end result is that the incompatibility of older people's needs with institutional cultures leads to both tacit and overt ageism within hospitals. Even the physical environment of the hospital can be hostile for older people. The burgeoning complexity of health care, with its myriad departments, clinics and technological installations, has resulted in confusing layouts, poor signage, lack of storage space and lack of day rooms – problems that impact especially on older people (Tadd et al., 2011).

Hospitals represent institutions in which ageist practices can flourish, not necessarily because of a wilful disregard for the feelings, rights and well-being of older people, but because the professional and organisational cultures within hospitals have developed from a model in which narrow tracts of expertise are deliberately cultivated. The cultivation of disease-specific expertise is advantageous to advancing the overall efficacy of clinical practices, but can engender an approach to patient care that is highly rationalised and instrumental, and which is not well adapted for patients who present with complex co-morbidities and additional emotional, psychological and social needs. This is not to deny the outstanding commitment, compassion and hard work of staff within the NHS, or the existence of many wards and hospitals in which older people do receive excellent care. Rather, I am suggesting that, where the rational scientific approach of modern medicine meets the messy and uncertain realities of elderly people in failing health, age-related discrimination is too often an unintended and unforeseen consequence.

'Bed blocking' and 'patient flow'

Forms of institutional and professional ageism within hospitals are crystallised in the discourse of 'bed blocking'. The term 'bed blocking' describes the occupation of an inpatient bed by a person who does not need the care that can be provided on the ward in which the bed is situated. It is taken by clinicians and hospital managers to be an illegitimate use of hospital resources that deprives other patients of access to the services that can be provided to the occupier of the bed. Though the term is not linguistically ageist, its underlying assumptions are rooted in the institutional cultures described above, which emphasise cure over care, to which elderly people's bodies may be unable to conform. Frequently, elderly hospital inpatients reach a point at which they no longer require the expertise of specialised clinicians, but cannot manage to return to their lives outside the hospital without additional support. It is at this point that hospital systems demand that they must be transferred to social care providers, with any delay in this transfer of care and responsibility regarded as an unwelcome interruption of the hospital's flow of patients. Contemporary management systems within hospitals define and record any delayed transfers of care, with power to define a patient's readiness for discharge regarded as the exclusive preserve of clinicians (Manzano-Santaella, 2010). Legitimacy of bed occupation rests on medical need alone, therefore.

The patient-blaming tone of the phrase 'bed blocking' has widely been replaced within health organisations with the term 'delayed transfer of care' (DTOC), which will be used in this book. Underlying the discourse, whether 'bed-blocking' or 'DTOC' is the preferred term, is a shared understanding among clinicians and hospital managers that each hospital bed's essence is as a tool in the treatment and management of a particular medical condition, rather than as the rightful temporary preserve of an individual person. Individual patients are expected by hospitals to 'flow' through their various compartments, in which differing clinical tasks can be undertaken. For example, a patient is a legitimate occupant of a bed on a surgical ward only for the purpose of preparation for, and recovery from, surgery. If a different medical need hinders the patient's discharge from hospital following recovery from surgery (for example an individual who contracts a serious respiratory infection following orthopaedic surgery), it would be expected that a bed on a different ward should be found (Benson et al., 2006). Thus, patients are treated as objects transferable to different centres of care, depending on the needs they present.

The system is not designed in this way deliberately to be inhumane. It represents a highly efficient way of organising and distributing expert clinical knowledge, with the purpose of ensuring that each individual person who is treated in hospital receives the best possible care and has the best chance of a satisfactory outcome. Indeed, it has long been acknowledged that prolonged stays in hospital are associated with a wide range of additional troubles for the patient, including increased risk of infections, pressure sores, deep vein thrombosis and loss of muscle condition leading to decreased mobility (Hirsch et al., 1990). Maintaining patients' 'flow' through the hospital is therefore important both to ensure that each hospital department can provide services as efficiently as possible and to ensure the best outcome for patients. The problem for older people is that often they cannot 'flow' through the hospital in the desired way because of the medical complexities their bodies present, and the social needs that arise from age-associated deteriorations of body and mind.

Clinicians make clear distinctions between medical needs, which are legitimate claimants of their time and resources, and social needs, which are held to be the preserve of other organisations and professionals (Latimer, 2000). Responsibility for delays caused by social needs is therefore, naturally, held by clinicians to be the responsibility of those other organisations. Since the 1990s, the medical profession, with its powerful voice in shaping public opinion and political discourse, has developed a narrative in which the dominant explanation for the occurrence of delayed transfers of care is that local authorities fail to provide the social care services for which they are responsible (Gill and Ingman, 1994). This is an incomplete understanding of the reasons for delayed transfers of care. Though variables related to social care have been shown to be strong predictors for delays (Challis et al., 2014), internal hospital factors (e.g. waiting on a specialist ward for services from another medical discipline) and an undersupply of rehabilitation services are also important factors (Glasby and Lester, 2004). For the period of 2018–2019, NHS England (2019) found that 28.9% of delayed transfers of care could be attributed to social care alone, with 9.2% attributable to both the NHS and social care services, and 61.9% attributable to the NHS alone. The evidence for the numbers of delayed transfers of care attributable to social care services is regularly a matter for dispute. During the fieldwork undertaken for this book, I observed daily meetings between social workers and a patient flow manager in which social workers corrected wrongly attributed records of delayed patient discharges on the hospital database. Attributing blame for a delayed transfer of care to an organisation outside the NHS appears helpful to ward managers' presentation of performance indicators, since length of patient stay is widely taken as a proxy measure for the efficiency of hospitals (Manzano-Santaella, 2010).

Despite the fact that the majority of delayed transfers of care are caused by internal factors within the NHS, the narrative of blame upon social care services became so widely accepted that, in 2003, the UK government passed the Community Care (Delayed Discharge) Act, which legislated for hospitals to be able to charge local authorities if they failed to provide services required for a discharge within forty eight hours of notification. Pitching services against each other in this way supports a false dichotomy between health and social care services when often both are of equal importance in meeting the needs of older people in ill health (Glasby, 2003). Though charging of local authorities has subsequently been made optional, local authorities in England and Wales nonetheless retain delayed transfers of care as an important key performance indicator for their social services. This embeds within social services departments an acceptance of the legitimacy of the 'patient flow' model and affirms that discharge planning must be the primary role for hospital social workers. It also discourages a holistic approach to older people as hospital inpatients that might be more appropriate where their physiological, psychological and social needs cannot be disaggregated.

The 'patient flow' model represents an efficient way to manage scarce resources and distribute expert clinical knowledge and skill, but can result in experiences of hospital for older people that are disorientating, disempowering and even humiliating. Older patients who cannot 'flow' through the hospital in the way the system demands may find that they are moved in and out of wards, and in and out of bays within wards, at all hours of the day and night (Tadd et al., 2011). As I observed during the fieldwork for this book, they may experience pressure from hospital staff to accept permanent placement in a residential care setting before they are emotionally ready to take such a significant life transition, or may be discharged to their homes reliant upon outdated formal care plans that are not adequate for their new needs, or upon informal carers who are unprepared for additional responsibilities. The prioritisation of efficiency relegates concern for the patient's humanity to a secondary issue and encourages neglect of patients' psychological and social needs.

Discharge planning as social work

Discharge planning, which can be understood as the primary activity of hospital social workers, occurs at the point when the hospital's systems demand that a patient moves on from the bed s/he is occupying. The hospital's system values speed above all other considerations, but good discharge planning takes time. Essential to the successful discharge of older patients whose health is vulnerable is a holistic approach in which complexities and uncertainties are thoroughly addressed. Social workers in hospital settings therefore frequently find that their aims and values conflict with the institutional system of which they are a part.

A typical discharge planning 'case' for a hospital social worker begins with a referral from a ward. Social work teams will usually not accept a patient for discharge planning until he/she is considered medically fit for discharge because the patient's presenting needs can change so much over the course of an admission. For example, there may be confusion or reduced mobility during the earlier part of the admission that resolves by the time the patient is no longer in need of inpatient care. The reluctance of social work teams to begin assessment until the patient is considered medically fit for discharge is an immediate cause of tension between social work departments and wards, because the time taken by social workers to carry out assessment is counted within the hospital's system as a delayed transfer of care. There is usually a waiting list for allocation of patients, causing a delay in the commencement of assessment of a day or two. Social work teams frequently receive referrals for patients who are not medically fit, as wards attempt to avoid delays and start up the process of social work assessment as soon as possible, and therefore must filter out some referrals in the early stages of assessment.

For a patient who is medically fit for discharge, the social work role involves co-ordinating information from clinicians within the hospital including doctors, nurses, occupational therapists, physiotherapists and speech and language therapists. Alongside this, social workers spend time with patients to find out what they want to happen, and time talking to the patient's family and carers. There are often disagreements between the different parties to be resolved. For example, the patient might wish to return to their own home, while clinicians may recommend levels of care that would require a residential placement and concerned family members might be pressing for a plan that minimises risk. The social work role often involves providing advocacy and brokering agreement regarding the discharge plan. Once a plan has been agreed, it must be sent to local authority managers for approval, and then services are arranged.

Many hospital social work teams do not review the care plans after discharge, but pass over that responsibility to community-based teams.

Some patients leaving hospital have complex ongoing health issues and may therefore be entitled to Continuing Healthcare funding (CHC) through the NHS. Whereas the social care services provided by local authorities are means-tested (with the exception of personal care services in Scotland), CHC is a non-means-tested provision. Through CHC, individuals may receive services through residential care or in the community. Assessment of needs is organised under the following categories (NHS, 2018b):

- breathing
- nutrition
- continence
- skin
- mobility
- communication
- psychological and emotional needs
- cognition (understanding)
- behaviour
- drug therapies and medication
- altered states of consciousness
- other significant care needs

An individual's needs under each category must be ranked 'priority', 'severe', 'high', 'moderate', 'low' or 'no needs'. In order to qualify for CHC, it must be agreed that a patient has at least one 'priority' need or at least two 'severe' needs. Eligibility can also be agreed if there is one 'severe' need and several other needs, or even simply a high number of complex and unpredictable needs. There is a great deal of room for interpretation and CHC-related decisions can vary widely depending not only on the health authority in which the assessment is conducted, but even between teams (Public Accounts Committee, 2018). Assessments for CHC must be agreed jointly by clinicians and representatives of the local authority, meaning that they are a regular task for hospital social workers and can be the source of disagreement and frustration (see Part II for further discussion). Social workers' contribution to the process is to make an assessment and to attend the multi-disciplinary meetings in which agreements must be reached. Where CHC is granted, responsibility for the care plan is transferred to clinicians – usually nurses. If CHC is not granted, social workers are responsible for arranging a care plan that will be administered by the local authority instead.

A source of complexity in hospital social work is the issue of patients' mental capacity, with around a quarter of all hospital beds occupied by people with dementia (Lakey, 2009). The hospital social workers involved in the research for this book all agreed that a high proportion of the patients referred to them had some level of impairment to cognition. Under the Mental Capacity Act 2005, assessment of mental capacity involves a two-stage test: there must be a formal diagnosis of a condition that disturbs the functioning of the mind, and it must be established that the person's ability to make a particular decision is impaired. Where a person is deemed not to be able to make a decision due to impaired mental capacity, the legislation requires that a decision must be taken in her/his best interests by family members and/or relevant professions. Social workers are often involved in the assessment of capacity and play a leading role in care planning where it is established that a person cannot make her/his own decision regarding care and living arrangements. As will be explored further in Part II, complexities arise in relation to the management of disagreements among the interested parties over individual patients' capacity and their best interests.

Critical gerontology and social work

Since hospital social work is concerned primarily with preparing for the reintegration of an elderly patient in the world outside the hospital, it is essential to discuss not only how older people are treated within hospitals, but how they take their place within wider society. The 'ageing population' is frequently cast as an intractable problem that impacts upon both the public and private spheres of life. In the public sphere, there is concern that older people's claim to the state's resources, both in the form of pensions and through the provision of health and social care services, places strain on the economy and appropriates the wealth of younger generations (Hastings and Rogowski, 2015). Similarly, in the private sphere, the reliance of older people on family members to provide care is often portrayed as having a detrimental impact on the health, wealth and happiness of younger generations (Walker, 2012). In other words, older people are seen in much of the popular discourse as a burden upon younger generations, and the increase in the number of people living into old age is understood not as an indicator of our good fortune, but rather as a troubling side effect of our contemporary social order that must be managed in some way. It is ironic that a social order that has produced such an unprecedented increase in longevity should, at least in the UK, be so inimical to the forms of social organisation necessary to make life in old age pleasant, or even tolerable.

Social work with older people tends to be valued less highly than social work with children and families (Lymbery, 2005) because social workers have held a long-standing perception that there are fewer opportunities for therapeutic or emancipatory practice with older people than with other groups (Stevenson, 1977). This low general esteem for the work is reflected in the lack of consideration for gerontology in social work education. Ageing is seldom explored in detail on qualifying courses and there is a wider disconnect between social work and gerontological research (Ray et al., 2009). Social work journals tend to cover policy issues related to older people but rarely address practice issues (Richards et al., 2014). Some social work practitioners are themselves guilty of colluding in ageism (Payne, 2012), whether through failing to challenge ageist assumptions within families or through their low expectations of the quality of life older people can expect. While reaching a certain age does not automatically mean that an individual is in need of social work, ageing often brings infirmities of physical and mental health that may create a need for social work (Lishman et al., 2018). The increasing size of the ageing population therefore represents an opportunity for social work to develop critical practices that can enhance older people's well-being, address inequalities and provide therapeutic interventions at an individual and/or family level (Ray et al., 2015). Critical gerontology has much to offer social work with older people, since it provides analysis of the way that many of the difficulties facing older people come about not as the inevitable consequence of bodily ageing, or of individual life choices, but through the operation of wider social and structural forces (Phillipson and Walker, 1987; Baars, 1991).

Hospital inpatients tend to encounter hospital social workers (HSWs) at a time in their life when they are experiencing a marked, irreversible decline in their health for the first time, or a significant progression of an ongoing decline in their health. This means that HSWs generally work with people who are transitioning into, or are already well-established in, the 'fourth age' – a normative state of advanced old age marked by physical and mental decline (Laslett, 1989; Baltes, 1997; Baltes and Smith, 1999). The fourth age can be difficult to define because of the varied way in which ageing can affect people – definitions that rely simply on age thresholds or even levels of impairment fail because they do not take account of their meaning within each individual's life (Grenier, 2012). While the term 'fourth age' can be used in clinical terms to denote a complex co-occurrence of disease and impairment in old age (Rockwood and Mitniski, 2007), its implications go beyond the individual experience of morbidity. It is perhaps best understood through contrast with notions of the 'third age' from which it emerged (Laslett, 1989). The concept of the third age revolves around active ageing – the continuing participation of older people in social life after retirement – constructing old age as a time of continued participation and citizenship, as opposed to withdrawal and adjustment to diminished status (Deeming, 2009). By contrast, the fourth age is associated with deficit, burden, weakness and dependence (Grenier, 2007; Pickard, 2016), and by implication a reduction in participation and agency. While positive portrayals of the third age have challenged discriminatory assumptions about old age as a time of withdrawal and decline, they have also been criticised for the polarisation between the active and healthy period of earlier old age and the stigma of decline commonly associated with advanced old age (Grenier, 2007). The concept of the third age therefore delays the marginalisation of elderly people, rather than preventing it altogether (Grenier, 2012).

Whereas the third age is distinguished as a period of freedom and self-definition, the fourth age is associated with a loss of individuality and agency brought about by dependence on others (Grenier and Phillipson, 2013). The fourth age therefore has significant cultural meaning as a 'social imaginary' (Gilleard and Higgs, 2010) in which personhood is lost and potential is void.

People in the fourth age are seen as having lost the ability to enact the power, status and citizenship roles of the third age and instead lose control through the physical and mental impairments that arise in advanced old age (Phillipson, 2013). This social imaginary allows for the 'othering' of older people, imposing upon them both alienation and vulnerability (Gilleard and Higgs, 2011a). The alienation of people in the fourth age is linked to their proximity to death – their impairments are seen less as disabilities which can be adjusted to, and rather as markers of a decline that is inexorable and indicative of imminent extinction (Grenier, 2012).

The boundary of the fourth age is marked out by frailty (Gilleard and Higgs, 2011b), which can be understood as both a state of bodily/mental weakness and as a state of high potential for morbidity (Degnen, 2007). The experience of frailty by older people is non-linear, involving both gradual decline and sudden change events, along with periods of stability (Skillbeck et al., 2018). Grenier (2007) argues that frailty can be conceived of as a 'dividing practice' (Foucault, 1982) in which the subject experiences objectification through being divided within her/himself or divided from others. A condition of frailty is seen as the opposite to healthy life and a failure to be engaged in active ageing (Grenier et al., 2017). As a dividing practice, the categorisation of frailty can be used to plan clinical services and to assess eligibility for social care services (Grenier, 2007). There is a risk, however, that frailty can become a 'black hole' in which the self of earlier life stages is lost and never to return (Gilleard and Higgs, 2010). Frailty has such destructive power over the self because of its nebulous status – it is neither a cultural identity nor a stable social position, meaning that opportunities for de-stigmatisation or protest against marginalisation are not available (Higgs and Gilleard, 2014). Indeed, Grenier et al. (2017) have argued that frailty comprises a status that has parallels both with Standing's (2010) conception of precarity as a position of vulnerability and insecurity within the labour market, and with Butler's (2009) conception of precarity as a politically induced position brought about by failing mechanisms of care and support. Thus, many frail people also live in a condition of insecure dependence, in which vulnerability in old age is amplified by disadvantage across the life course and underpinned by marginalisation, stigma and othering.

While frailty can be seen as a uniquely disempowering category that is destructive of personhood and agency, critical gerontology has begun to point to approaches that offer liberation for people in the fourth age. In contrast to Gilleard and Higgs' (2010) view of frailty as a black hole of unbecoming in which agency is not possible, Grenier and Phillipson (2013) argue that an expanded understanding of how agency may be enacted can challenge the polarisation between health and frailty. While the exercise or even expression of deliberate choice may be constrained by physical or mental impairment, and individual or collective action to produce change may not be possible, acts of verbal or non-verbal communication may represent forms of expression that should not be assumed to be lacking all agency. A conception of personhood is therefore required that focuses less on the value of a person based on her/his ability to exercise individual action or intentionality, and more on each person's intrinsic worth as a member of the wider collective of human life (Grenier et al., 2017). This can be seen, for example, in new approaches to working with people with dementia that are founded upon an understanding of the self as interactional and inter-embodied rather than purely individual, and challenge assumptions that people with dementia are purely receivers of care with nothing to contribute to those around them (Jenkins, 2014).

For social work, critical gerontology offers a critique of the active ageing policies that are aimed at reducing reliance on state services and devalue those who have become frail and vulnerable (Lloyd et al., 2014). The emphasis on personalisation in English social care, for example, has the effect of reinforcing the message of individual responsibility on those experiencing the most need, who are least equipped for self-help (Ray and Phillips, 2012). Social workers need to be aware that, when tasked with assessing the needs of older people for care, they are not only working with people who have social and bodily needs arising from physical and mental impairment, but people who are moving into a period of life marked by marginalisation, discrimination and stigma (Ray et al., 2015). The older people whom social workers encounter are in need of more than simple care management – they need assistance to challenge the blame for their need that is placed on them by policy-makers and even their carers (Lloyd et al., 2014), relational work that can take account of their life history and help them through significant transitions (Phillips and Waterson, 2005) and assistance with complex family situations (Statham et al., 2006). Social work with older people often involves negotiating the interplay between family dynamics, the cumulative effects of disadvantage and the ever-present influence of ageism (Richards et al., 2014). Carrying out these tasks effectively requires social workers to develop expertise in working with older people, through both engagement with gerontological theory and developing specialist skills for communicating and building relationships with older people who are affected by dementia and cognitive decline (Richards et al., 2014).

While there is potential, or at least a need, for a critical gerontological practice to emerge in social work, the community care system is not a fertile ground for its development. Community care discourages social workers from engagement in relational work with older people, placing little value on older people's narratives and offering little space for working with people to address psychosocial issues arising from their transitions through the life course (Sullivan, 2009). The social work value base, however, does place heavy emphasis on promoting human rights and social justice, while social work's knowledge base is centred upon understanding the individual within her/his socio-political context (Ray et al., 2015). Social work is therefore well equipped to develop to meet the needs of a growing ageing population, but will only be able to do so if it can expand its practices beyond the narrow individual focus of care management. For this to occur, social work needs to advocate for its right to develop its role with older people, drawing on both critical gerontological theory and an increasing base of empirical research. In hospital social work, critical gerontological approaches have the potential to enhance the practices undertaken by HSWs in the process of making discharge plans and may also inform new developments in relation to supporting people to change and sustain health-protective behaviours.

Social work and liquid modernity

While critical gerontology emphasises the importance of understanding the influence of wider social systems and structures in the lives of older people, it is important to acknowledge that hospital social work is heavily focused on intervention at the individual level only. As will be discussed in the following chapters, the dominance of the care management model over social work with older people is underpinned by the economic and political ideology of neoliberalism, which extols market discipline and consumer choice as the most efficient means of organising public services (Griffiths Report, 1988). The hegemony of neoliberalism over policy-making in the UK since the Thatcher era is matched by a wider and pervasive spread of individualisation in the way our lives are led, which has particular significance for gerontological social work. Bauman's (2000a) concept of liquid modernity is helpful in making sense of the spread and extent of individualisation and its importance for social work. Bauman coined the term 'liquid modernity' to describe the most recent development of the modern era, in which the old certainties of 'solid' modernity have been replaced by instability, ambivalence and impermanence, all of which are driven by rampant individualism. Whereas the era of 'solid modernity' was characterised by routine and compliance – exemplified in the institution of the Fordist factory – liquid modernity casts each individual as both free and responsible for her/his own being. Bauman argues that liquid modernity represents an inescapable fate in which the individual is responsible for her/himself without having the power to control events. The comforts of permanent employment, insoluble life partnerships and collective responsibilities have been replaced by globalised markets, intolerance of imperfections and individual human rights that protect difference rather than solidarity.

In Bauman's understanding of liquid modernity, a consequence of individualisation and the relaxing of social norms and traditions is that each individual moves from life project to life project throughout their lives, since

> [t]he pain which used to be caused by unduly limited choice has now been replaced by no less a pain – though this time the pain is caused by an obligation to choose without trusting the choices made and without confidence that further choices will bring the target any closer.
>
> (Bauman, 2007, p. 106)

Giddens also notes the openness of choices presented by the contemporary world, but optimistically interprets this as a chance for each person to participate in 'life politics' in which each person has a chance to shape their own world as they choose (Giddens, 1992; Giddens, 1999). As Garrett (2004) notes, however, for many of the people whom social workers encounter, the idea of life politics is illusory, since inequality and oppression remain deeply embedded in their lives, with tradition and habit still serving to keep people from exercising absolute freedom of choice. For many older people with whom social workers are concerned, social conventions may still have a power that is absent for younger generations, and the social work task may therefore involve liberation through challenging restrictive norms. Where older people are engaged in life politics and the assumption of individual responsibility for their lives, the physical and mental health challenges that old age often presents, combined with age-based discrimination, may nonetheless have a crushing impact. Thus, social workers need to have a regard for the disruptions of individual freedom that older people encounter.

Despite his advancing years, Bauman gave little attention to the issues of old age while writing about liquid modernity. It is not difficult to see how the human needs that older people's social workers regularly encounter fit Bauman's description of liquid modernity, however. The uncertainty characteristic of liquid modernity can be seen in the lives of the older people with whom social workers are concerned – indeed, as noted above, the fourth age has been said to be characterised by the precarity that Bauman places at the heart of his conception (Grenier et al., 2017). The advances in medical care and associated increases in life expectancy noted above have led to a situation in which increasing numbers of older people are living for long periods with chronic illnesses, increasing disability and progressing frailty (Age UK, 2017). This means that the life course for many people of advanced years has become more complex and less predictable. Illnesses particularly associated with old age, e.g. various forms of dementia and Parkinson's disease, can progress in a variety of ways and may result in physical, psychological and emotional states that are difficult to anticipate (Barry and Yuill, 2016). Similarly, rates of cancer survival are increasing, yet survival of cancer often brings with it ongoing complex medical needs (Macmillan, 2014). The same can be said of survival of heart attacks and strokes (Johansson et al., 2017; Greenwood and McKenzie, 2010). During the era of solid modernity, numbers of people living with chronic illness were lower and the association between morbidity and mortality in old age was closer. The increase in survival of disease among older people, while of course welcome, has brought with it a new uncertainty for older people about the course their lives will take.

Living with chronic illness in old age brings with it a number of consequences that reflect the uncertainty of the liquid modern era. Aspects of the social order may become reversed, e.g. while more women than men act as informal carers overall, among the over 70s, a higher proportion of men than women are carers – usually husbands caring for their spouses (Dahlberg et al., 2007). The development of dementia in a life partner is likely eventually to change a spousal relationship from one of mutual support to one perceived as involving total responsibility on one side and total dependency on the other (Kitwood, 1997).

Similarly, for older people who are cared for by their adult children, the nature of the relationship between parent and child is likely to be transformed by the development of a caring relationship (Plank et al., 2012). Thus, long-established ways of being for older people may have to be abandoned, and the nature of their relationships with the people closest to them may be profoundly and irreversibly altered. Living with chronic illness in old age becomes a liquid existence, in which all former certainties can be replaced with new and unpredictable ways of being.

Just as old age may be argued to have liquid qualities, elements of liquid modernity impact on older people in unique ways. The living environments of liquid modern societies continue to develop at a dizzying pace, with digital technology promoting means of communication from which older people may feel excluded (Hill et al., 2015) and urban redevelopment resulting in older people's home towns becoming unfamiliar to them (Phillips et al., 2011). The individualising nature of liquid modern times means that people are left with full responsibility for dealing with a fate over which they may have had little or no power (Bauman, 2000a). Within liquid modern society, this results in discriminatory attitudes towards older people, who are derided for being a 'burden' when they have care needs (Ray and Phillips, 2012; Hastings and Rogowski, 2015). People who are unable to maintain their own independence are blamed for their helplessness and contributions they make to their communities and families are not recognised (Lloyd et al., 2014), or their existence is pathologised as not worth living. Cultural representations of dementia, for example, present it as a fearful and tragic obliteration of personality (Hillman and Latimer, 2017), meaning that recognition of the personhood of older people is diminished.

The economic model of neoliberalism that underpins liquid modernity impacts on older people in need of care in two ways: state services are reduced to a minimum and targeted only at the highest need, which can result in lower, yet still substantial, needs being overlooked (Penna and O'Brien, 2013); and people of working age are required to be flexible workers who can relocate easily and commit additional hours to their job whenever required (Harvey, 2005), meaning that it is often extremely difficult for family members of working age to provide the care that their elderly relatives may need. This is not to say that younger generations are withdrawing from responsibility to care for their elders, but that family members are having to find new ways of managing their obligations towards one another (Bernard et al., 2001). Difficulties with the physical availability of family members to provide support are often particularly acute for older people in rural areas, which younger people are more likely to leave (Cloke et al., 1997).

It is possible, then, to denote the challenges faced by people in advanced old age in the contemporary era as 'liquid old age', which can be thought of as a state of precarious living caused by the uncertainties of unpredictably declining physical and/or mental health, within a society in which responsibility for one's welfare rests primarily with the individual, and in which the demands of the neoliberal economy limit access to state and family care. Issues of precarity and uncertainty are often to the fore in the lives of hospital inpatients as they approach discharge, since the availability of care is restricted by liquid modern living. Hospital social work has a role to play in addressing the challenges of liquid old age and social workers therefore need to take a critical approach to working with older people that includes addressing ageist assumptions and practices both among families and within their own occupational culture.

Conclusion

Social work is not simply the product of the will of practitioners but is naturally shaped by the socio-cultural context in which it occurs (Wallace and Pease, 2011). This means that hospital social work must necessarily be shaped by institutional and professional systems and cultures that are not well adapted to the realities and requirements of older people, and a society in which older people are frequently unvalued and stigmatised. Circumstances often conspire to disempower older people in hospitals, where powerful institutional systems, individual professionals and family members can all connect in ways that result in loss of dignity, agency and even sense of self. It is possible for social workers to choose how their practice is shaped by these contexts – whether they follow the path of complicity or resistance. There is potential for social work in hospitals to be a powerful force in countering age-related and other inter-sectional injustices that affect elderly hospital patients.

Notes

1 Around 11 per cent of the population have some form of private health insurance (King's Fund, 2014). See https://www.kingsfund.org.uk/sites/default/files/media/commission-appendix-uk-private-health-market.pdf.
2 I have chosen to use the word 'patient' to denote those in receipt of medical services with whom hospital social workers are involved, despite its connotations of subjugation to medical power, on the basis that being a medical patient is a universal experience that reflects our taking up of medical care as a citizenship right.
3 I use the term 'clinician' throughout to denote those who are involved directly in the medical care of hospital inpatients (e.g. doctors, nurses, physiotherapists, occupational therapists, etc.).

2 A brief history of hospital social work

Introduction

This chapter explores the historic development of hospital social work, from its nineteenth-century origins in the work of hospital almoners through to the recent contemporary era, in which the care management model is dominant. The story of hospital work is one of a rise and fall in terms of both its status within the wider occupation of social work and its standing among other occupational groupings within the hospital. Paying heed to the history of social work in hospitals is instructive because it reminds us of the currently unfulfilled potential social work has as a contributor to health care services, and because it contains lessons that must be understood if social work with older people in general is to advance itself beyond the primarily administrative purposes upon which it has been based since the advent of care management (Lymbery, 2005).

The neglect of hospital social work as a distinctive activity is stark in both the literature on the social history of medicine and in social work's own narratives of its development. Waddington (2011), for example, makes no mention at all of hospital social workers or almoners, while Porter (1999) overlooks the role of social workers in the development of public health care, other than to point out that the presence of almoners in hospitals in the early part of the twentieth century was useful to doctors in increasing their earning potential by ensuring that even the poor paid something towards their treatment. In the social work literature, research on hospital social work is relatively sparse. Standard social work text books (e.g. Wilson et al., 2012; Lishman et al., 2018) often divide social work into categories, such as 'children and families', 'adults with mental health problems', etc. but do not allot hospital social work a category of its own. When the historical contribution of hospital social work to the development of social work knowledge and approaches, and to the professionalisation of social work, is understood, such invisibility in the literature becomes troubling, reflecting perhaps an overall shrinking in the ambitions of social work as a force of change within society.

The origins of social work

While many human societies have taken measures to provide welfare for the vulnerable and have established a tradition of charity, social work is a unique response to the unprecedented social and cultural complexities of modernity (Webb, 2007). Until the beginning of the nineteenth century, the primary occupations for the common people of Britain were agriculture, domestic service and hand-loom weaving, a state of affairs that had remained substantially unchanged for many centuries (Burnett, 1994). The extraordinary advent of industrialisation, however, with its increasing use of mechanisation and mass manufacture, combined with repeated crises in agriculture in the first half of the nineteenth century, altered the common way of life in Britain forever, resulting in the migration and concentration in cities of unskilled labourers, whose living conditions were squalid (Royle, 2012). This upheaval brought about a generalised increase in anxiety and uncertainty, with old ideas and long-standing traditions called into question (Webb, 2007). Significantly, urbanisation created a new proximity of living spaces between rich and poor, with the result that the rich could not ignore the squalor of their neighbours. The threat of the congregated poor became of great concern, their destructive potential repeatedly demonstrated during the Luddite uprisings of 1811–1812, violent protests over electoral reform in 1831 and numerous other riots and uprisings (Royle, 2012). The terrifying example of the French Revolution meant that such convulsions could not be ignored.

A tradition of statutory poverty relief existed in Britain with the Elizabethan Poor Laws, which obliged local parishes to provide subsistence for those in absolute penury (Kidd, 1999). The Poor Law Amendment Act of 1834, however, reflected the inadequacy of such laws within the radically altered context of industrialisation. The aim of the new Poor Law, with its creation of workhouses for the destitute, was to centralise and standardise provision, while ensuring that receipt of poor relief was less attractive than self-help (Payne, 2005). This reflected an underlying ideology that poverty and unemployment were the result of individual inadequacy, rather than wider social forces (Lowe, 2004). In counterpoint to this ideology there persisted the Christian tradition of almsgiving, which often supplemented or replaced the relief provided by the Poor Laws, and working-class reform movements such as the Chartists and the Trade Unions, which aimed to improve the political representation of the poor (Payne, 2005).

Social work in Britain can trace its origins to two distinctive organisational strands of innovative responses of the wealthier classes to the deprivation of the urban poor in modernity: the Charity Organisation Society (COS) and the Settlement movement (Doel, 2012). The COS represented a reaction against the Christian tradition of giving alms indiscriminately to the poor as a religious exercise, which it asserted encouraged fecklessness and inhibited individuals' capacity to develop self-help (Payne, 2005). Rather, its members argued that a scientific method was required to discern whether recipients might use aid to re-establish independence or whether they would continue to rely on charity as an easier option than self-help (Shaw, 2008). For those latter, who would be classed as 'undeserving', the provisions of the Poor Laws were thought to be sufficient (Payne 2005). The primary method of intervention for the COS was individual casework, in which the circumstances of the applicant for charitable aid would be formally assessed using inductive investigation (Webb, 2007). While the deliberate discrimination between supposedly 'deserving' and 'undeserving' poor appears harsh and regressive to modern eyes, subjecting the poor to new forms of surveillance (Foucault, [1975] 1991) the COS had at its roots a humanitarian ambition to relieve the suffering caused by poverty (Seed, 1973). Indeed, the more humanitarian aspects of the casework approach grew to prominence through the first half of the twentieth century as the profession of social work formed. Under the influence of emerging psychodynamic theory, social workers would develop an increasingly therapeutic orientation, seeking to assist people to overcome their problems through understanding their psychological processes (Payne, 2005).

Whereas the COS argued that individual failings were the cause of poverty, and that through individual casework such failings were being directly addressed (Rooff, 1972), the Settlement movement based its actions on the understanding that inequalities and disadvantage were at the root of the perceived moral failings of the poor (Barnett and Barnett, 1915). Residential 'settlements' in deprived areas were therefore established, in which university graduates could share the benefits of education with poorer members of society (Reinders, 1982). For settlement workers, a heavy emphasis was placed on understanding the socio-economic causes of individual difficulty, while co-residence with the urban poor had the twin purposes of breaking down barriers and offering to the poor a positive moral example (Manthorpe, 2002). Whereas the COS focused their activities on individual casework, the Settlements' services tended to have a more communal emphasis, in the form of youth clubs, educational programmes, art exhibitions, drama societies and even country and seaside holidays for children (Matthews and Kimmis, 2001). There was also an emphasis on campaigning for change in social policy, based on an understanding that poverty was most frequently caused by social inequality and disadvantage, rather than individual personal failing (Payne, 2005). The social action approach to social work embodied by the Settlement movement became less prominent as social work developed through the twentieth century, aside from the brief rise of radical social work in the 1970s, but lives on through the work of non-governmental organisations, and continues to inform social work education and its underpinning values.

The existence of two originating organisations with opposing values can lead to the conclusion that social work is composed of two working models that have always been, to some extent, in tension: individually orientated casework, and structurally orientated social action. As Lymbery (2005) notes, however, such a conclusion overlooks the importance of social administration as a third significant strand in the development of social work. While the work of the COS gave rise to the development of casework, administration of charitable resources was its ultimate aim. In current times, the individually orientated casework approach has come to dominate professional social work yet, as with the COS, this practice involves both therapeutic or reformative approaches at the individual level and the gatekeeping and distribution of resources. As will be seen, social administration is a particularly important part of the story of hospital social work's origins, and is central to the roles performed by social workers in hospitals.

The beginnings of hospital social work

Traditionally, medicine had been practised at a local, individual level, which required that a patient should pay the doctor directly for medical services, which were usually provided by the doctor visiting the patient's home. The rapid urbanisation of the early nineteenth century, however, led to a widespread establishment of new hospitals, which were financed either by individual philanthropy or public subscription (Porter, 1999). Some workers were able to join friendly societies or mutuals, which might fund the cost of medical treatment for them, if not their dependants (Gosden, 1961). For the majority of the urban poor, who could not afford to pay for a private consultation, however, access to medical care could only be obtained through the hospitals, and only if the patient was in possession of a letter of recommendation from a subscriber who had contributed significantly to the building and costs of the hospital (Simmons, 2005). Subscribers were limited in how many letters they could distribute, depending on the size of the contribution they had made, and therefore letters of recommendation were typically reserved for subscribers' employees. The first hospital that could be accessed without a subscriber's letter, the Royal Free Hospital, was established in London in 1828, and was followed by several more. The outpatients' departments of the free hospitals quickly became overcrowded and concern grew that the cause of overcrowding was the abuse of the free hospitals' charity by those who could afford to pay for treatment (Willmott, 1996). Hospital social work was therefore established at the instigation of the COS, with the intention of rooting out from the free clinics those who could afford to pay (Sackville, 1986). Despite a Select Committee report in 1893 arguing that abuse of the free hospitals was fairly limited, the general secretary of the COS, Charles Lock, recommended the creation of 'hospital almoner' posts, to investigate the circumstances of those seeking free medical care (Simmons, 2005). Thus, in 1895, Mary Stewart was appointed as the first Lady Almoner of the Royal Free Hospital, and hospital social work was born.

The integration of the early almoners into hospitals was not easy. Conflicts between almoners and doctors and nurses were common from the beginning (Moberly Bell, 1961; Butrym, 1967; Willmott, 1996), with clinicians seemingly resistant to allowing access to medical care to be to be decided and monitored by an outsider. Brewer and Lait (1980) argue that the resistance of clinicians towards the almoner's role was derived not only from a suspicion of outsiders to the hospital, but also from doubts about the knowledge claims of these early social workers and their competence over their chosen field.

Almoners quickly developed their practice to claim participation in curative actions, going beyond their initial purpose of assessing means to pay for treatment to seeking to ensure that patients would be able to maximise the benefit of their medical treatment (Willmott, 1996). Clinicians' resistance to the influence of almoners was much in evidence when almoners began to take an interest in work with expectant mothers and with tuberculosis patients (Moberly Bell, 1961), which was clearly beyond the mandate through which their posts had originally been established. The early almoners' ability to extend their role in the face of such resistance reflects their belief in the importance of addressing the social causes of disease, their determination to extend both their knowledge and competence, and their independence as agents within the hospital. Moberly Bell (1961) claims that the utility of the almoners was quickly demonstrated and that it was their visible success that helped them to become established in the face of clinicians' resistance, yet Brewer and Lait (1980) express doubt over the evidence for this, pointing out that the Royal Free Hospital refused to extend Mary Stewart's appointment beyond the agreed two years until additional funding was provided by the COS. The truth probably lies somewhere between these two poles: that the work of almoners was not revolutionary in its scope or success, but came to be valued by many clinicians working in the free hospitals who could not help but be aware of the squalor around them and the associated social problems experienced by many of their patients.

It is of interest that the occupation of almoner was, in its early years, so explicitly associated with female workers. Although it is documented that there was at least one male member of the Almoners' Committee in the early 1900s, male almoners were not common until after the Second World War (Sackville, 1989). This would cause a high attrition rate for almoners for much of the twentieth century, since many would give up their work or reduce their working hours following marriage and childbirth (Dedman, 1996). The early female domination of almoner posts reflects the influence of both the COS and the settlement movement in the development of the occupation. As a form of philanthropic work, much like other branches of the COS, the position of almoner offered an opportunity for young women of wealthier backgrounds to find occupation outside the home (Simmons, 2005). Preparation for such work could be found through the settlements, which began to represent a primitive form of professional training for social work (Parry and Parry, 1979). This perhaps explains why the early almoners, while maintaining strong links with the COS, quickly developed the role from being primarily focused on means assessment to assisting doctors to understand the social causes underlying disease and mobilising the appropriate resources to remedy destitution (Cullen, 2013). Such ambitions in Britain were enhanced by the pioneering work of the first almoner in the USA, Ida Cannon, who, with the support of the Chief of Medicine, Ethel Cohen, at Massachusetts General Hospital, argued that almoners could, and should, influence physicians (Cannon, 1913). It is possible that almoners' raising of physicians' awareness of the effects of environment on health contributed to the medical trend of convalescent homes and sanatoria in the early twentieth century. Indeed, arranging convalescent stays became a regular part of almoners' work at this time (Sackville, 1986). This suggests a clear link with the practice of settlements in providing holidays for children.

While early social workers might be influenced by the thinking of either the COS or the settlements, they of course would begin to form their own opinions based on the situations they encountered. The first almoner's appointment through the COS might suggest a resolute belief in thrift and self-help (Willmott, 1996), yet in fact she accepted a large majority of patients she assessed – around 70 per cent – for free help and also referred them onto other charities for further assistance (Cullen, 2013). The interest in supporting patients to ensure that they were able to take the maximum possible benefit from their treatment ensured that the work of the almoner quickly became a practice which can be recognised as 'social work'. Over the ensuing decades, almoners were challenged with responding to the social needs arising from new forms of medical treatment, including psychiatry, as well as new forms of need, such as work with the wounded of the First World War and coping with the epidemic of sexually transmitted disease that accompanied the war (Sackville, 1986). This interest was echoed in the aftermath of the Second World War, when almoners recognised the social impact of sexually transmitted diseases and argued that they were best placed to help both sufferers and their spouses because of their unique social and psychological understanding (Manchée, 1945).

Significantly, hospital social work was the first branch of social work in the UK to attempt to professionalise, with the establishment of a professional organisation, professional training and professional registration early in the twentieth century (Payne, 2005). Their day-to-day close proximity to other, more established, occupational groups may have been influential in encouraging almoners to seek professionalisation through this means. The Almoners' Committee was formed in 1903 and quickly asserted independent but friendly relations with the COS, which remained responsible for the selection and training of almoners (Sackville, 1986). A dispute between the Almoners' Committee and the COS during 1906–1907, however, resulted in a second independent body, the Almoners' Council, being set up to oversee almoner selection and education (Sackville, 1986). The two separate bodies would not merge until the end of the second world war, though by this time the Almoners' Council had reconstituted itself as the Hospital Almoners Association, and the Almoners' Council as the Institute of Hospital Almoners. The emergence of these professional bodies is indicative of an ambition for the specialised knowledge and skills of almoners to be recognised alongside those of clinicians and to gain the benefits of power and social closure provided by professional status (Friedson, 1970).

The training of almoners involved a period of six months spent in the offices of the COS, learning about the difficulties experienced by the poor and the avenues of support available, and developing practical skills related to making home visits and writing letters. Six months of studying sociology within a university was also required. After this, an internship within an almoners' office would be completed before a candidate could then be considered for an almoner's post (Kemp, 1912). Trainee almoners were taught about the hierarchies of hospitals but, while a sense of respect for consultant physicians as having ultimate responsibility for the patient's wellbeing was fostered, they were expected to stand as independent caseworkers, rather than simply providers of an ancillary service (Loxley, 1996). The professionalisation of almoners may have been driven by the close association between social problems and help-seeking at free hospitals, inasmuch as they presented an opportunity for almoners to perform 'social diagnosis' and expert treatment (Cullen, 2013). Such claims are significant, since occupations offering personal services often place emphasis on their curative role, at the expense of caring duties, when attempting to establish professional status (Hugman, 1991). Rashid's (2000) argument that the curative or rescuing elements of social work practice are more appropriately conceptualised as vocational than as professional overlooks the presence of altruistic aims in all occupations that aspire to professional status. In other words, all professions could be interpreted as vocations.

If almoners saw it as their primary, professional function to provide material and therapeutic support to patients, their association with assisting hospitals with assessing the financial circumstances of patients was nonetheless resolutely maintained (Willmott, 1996). Moreover, from the 1920s onwards, almoners accepted responsibility for more formal assessment of patients' means, so that they would determine the charges applicable to patients in charitable hospitals and public infirmaries (Lymbery, 2005). The desire to maintain such an administrative function in the midst of a deliberate project of professionalisation perhaps indicates that the social work of almoners was not yet accepted as an indispensable part of hospital treatment. Almoners were at times resentful of their administrative duties, arguing that these took them away from the more complex and interesting work for which they had expertise (e.g. Manchée, 1944, in Lymbery, 2005). By 1943, however, the position of almoners was strong enough that the Royal College of Physicians recommended that all hospitals should employ qualified almoners – both to work with patients and to contribute to medical education (Dedman, 1996).

The involvement of almoners (later called medical social workers) in the education of doctors and nurses has been taken by some writers (e.g. Moberly Bell, 1961; Butrym, 1967) to be confirmation of their relatively high status. It should be recognised, however, that this contribution was far from systematic. Butrym (1967) admitted that the extent of medical social workers' involvement as teachers on medical and nursing courses varied depending on the priority individual schools placed on the incorporation of social sciences, and bemoaned the lack of involvement of social workers in planning the social medicine curriculum. Similarly, Manchée's (1944) description of the contribution of almoners to medical education suggests that it was limited to one-off talks and demonstrations, although she also notes that almoners would contribute explanations of patients' social circumstances during medical rounds. The significance of this latter contribution is difficult to estimate, but suggests that almoners were at least able to keep the social causes of illness on the medical agenda. Despite almoners' contributions, the Todd Report of 1968 identified a general deficit in medical students' training in the behavioural sciences, which resulted in the formal incorporation of psychology and sociology, delivered by academics from those disciplines, within the medical curriculum. The arrival of sociologists and psychologists reduced the need for, and recognition of, teaching by almoners in medical education and the contribution of social work is now entirely overlooked in the sociology of medicine (e.g. see Scambler, 2009). Overall, the contribution of social work to medical education cannot be thought of as more than piecemeal and sporadic.

From the NHS to the Seebohm Report: the medical social workers

The introduction of the NHS in 1948 represented both a challenge and a threat to almoners. Abolition of charges for hospital care meant that they were at last liberated from the administrative duties that they so resented. Their role was not well understood by the public or by other professionals (Dedman, 1996), which meant that there was danger of their being overlooked in the planning of new services, but also potential for them to expand the scope of their duties and practice. The creation of posts related to public health, such as health visitors, posed a threat to almoners' position, both because of the possible overlap of duties and because doctors could ask health visitors to carry out home visits without involving the almoner (Sackville, 1987). During this period, however, almoners won two symbolic battles that enhanced their status as an occupational group. The first was that they successfully resisted being registered as 'Professions Auxiliary to Medicine' in favour of the less subordinate 'Non-medical Professional and Technical Staff' (Dedman, 1996). The second was successful resistance to the proposal that non-qualified workers could do the job of almoners in hospitals in which no qualified almoner was present (Sackville, 1987). While some unqualified workers were accepted to work under the direction of qualified staff, acknowledgement of the need for almoners to have a recognised qualification enhanced their claim to professional status.

With the abolition of the association with assessing financial means, the title of 'almoner' fell out of favour, and the Institute of Almoners formally changed its name to the Institute of Medical Social Workers in 1964. Although medical social workers had defended their status and role in the early years of the NHS, by the 1960s, the sheer size of the organisation and its need to reorganise left medical social workers' interests marginalised (Sackville, 1987). Consciousness was growing of the fragmentary nature of social work services and the idea of having a unified professional organisation to represent all social workers ran alongside the growing attraction of integrated social services departments (Payne, 2002). The majority of medical social workers would vote to amalgamate the Institute of Medical Social Workers with other social work associations as the British Association of Social Workers (BASW) at the end of that decade (Dedman, 1996). The willingness of medical social workers to disband their professional association is surprising in view of how highly contested their professional organisation had been from the outset. Their willingness at the end of the 1960s to merge identities with other branches of social work suggests that medical social workers had lost confidence in their status as a discrete professional grouping. No doubt the downgrading of their teaching role within medical education following the Todd Report (1968) contributed further to their sense of waning professional status and influence.

Despite medical social workers' willingness to embrace a generic social work identity, they did not fit automatically into the local authority social services departments that were created on the recommendation of the Seebohm Report (1968) and were not included in the Local Authority Social Services Act 1970. This did not deter the Institute of Medical Social Workers from formally amal-gamating with BASW, however, and medical social workers were initially active and influential, for example ensuring that only qualified social workers would be eligible to join the association (Payne, 2002). The generic social services depart-ments of the 1970s offered social work a protected sphere of practice and control and, in these terms, appeared to promise recognised professional status (Payne, 2005). Social work's progress towards professional status, however, was impeded both by the ambiguity of its knowledge base (Brewer and Lait, 1980) and by its own ambivalence about whether professional status is even desirable (Stevenson, 2005). Belief in the altruistic and useful function of professions was brought into question by critiques of professionalism as serving the ambitions of professionals rather than the people who require their services (e.g. Johnson, 1972; Larson 1977; Illich et al., 1977). The requirement of qualification for membership was abandoned in 1975, both because of a radical critique of professional elitism and because of the pressure from members for BASW to pursue improvements in pay and working conditions, which required a more inclusive membership base (Payne, 2002). Thus, the ambition for professional status that had characterised medical social work's earlier emergence was lost within the wider development of social work's identity.

When medical social work teams finally joined local authority social ser-vices departments in 1974, they quickly found that they were placed under pressure to give their time to other parts of the service and their branch of social work became perceived by colleagues as an easier option (Osborn, 1996). The full ramifications of accepting local authority employment may not have been apparent at the time, but would have a profound and perma-nent effect on the profession in the decades to come. For now, however, if medical social work did lose some of its prestige after the Seebohm reforms, the location of teams of social workers within hospitals was not affected, and medical social workers could be sure of their acceptance as legitimate mem-bers of the hospital's professional order – as symbolised by their wearing of white coats while on duty (Rushton and Davies, 1984). Numbers of social workers based in hospitals grew steadily from the mid-1970s to the mid-1980s and it was recognised that hospital social work departments offered high quality services for patients and also had the benefit of being cost-effective

(Connor and Tibbitt, 1988). The genericism instituted by the Seebohm Report meant that hospital-based social workers' roles expanded to include child protection, with medical social workers taking responsibility for responding in cases in which injuries to a child treated by the hospital were the first indication of concern. Other roles included assessing women who were seeking the termination of pregnancy and providing services to new families identified as vulnerable through the midwifery services. The assessment of women for pregnancy terminations by social workers was not required by the Abortion Act 1967; the act required rather that two doctors should agree on the grounds for permitting each procedure. However, reports by medical social workers on the social circumstances of women became central to many doctors' willingness to certify that continuation of the pregnancy would cause the mother's mental health grave injury.

Hospital social work and community care

At the end of the 1980s, hospital social work represented a varied area of practice in which social workers had scope to perform both therapeutic and practical/administrative roles for a wide range of people. Various structures existed for hospital social workers: in some hospitals, social worker posts were formally attached to particular units or specialisms (e.g. paediatrics, cardiology etc.), yet in others, teams would provide services across medical disciplines (Rushton and Davies, 1984). Hospital social workers' regular functions included counselling patients to come to terms with their illness, liaising with patients' families, applying for charitable grants on patients' behalf and carrying out the statutory functions required by local authorities. The introduction of the NHS and Community Care Act 1990, however, transformed mainstream hospital social work[1] into a practice solely focused upon needs assessment and discharge planning for patients who were too vulnerable to return home without new care arrangements, but who did not require ongoing inpatient medical care. Most influential over hospital social work was the legislation's new requirement that all people going into residential care must be assessed by a qualified social worker. This dramatically increased the number of assessments required of hospital social workers, with the result that other roles were quickly dispensed with, and hospital social workers' ability to do any work other than discharge planning was drastically curtailed (Rachman, 1997). Other than in mental health work, the therapeutic roles that adults' social workers in general had laid claim to were vastly diminished by the new legislation (Sullivan, 2009), and hospital social work, in particular, became an occupation much more closely associated with social administration.

Along with the Children Act 1989, the passing of the NHS and Community Care Act was a defining moment in UK social policy, since these two pieces of legislation marked the end of an ambition for universal services that was the hallmark of the post-war welfare state. This ambition was replaced by a new emphasis on targeting statutory services where need and risk were most obvious (Lymbery, 2001). The intention behind the NHS and Community Care Act 1990 was to encourage provision of social care services by private enterprises, which could be purchased by a local authority on behalf of citizens in need (McDonald, 2006). The role of social workers within this system would be to assess the need and eligibility of individuals for services, and to assist in making arrangements for those services to be delivered by a third party. This type of work, especially for hospital social workers, tended to focus on elderly people, whose care arrangements had often been left to unqualified workers to manage prior to the new legislation (Lymbery, 2005). Imposition of the care planning role is often understood to have brought about a de-skilling and de-professionalisation of social work with adults (Dustin, 2007; Lymbery and Postle, 2015), since it places less emphasis on the relational skills of the social worker, who is required only to find out the person's needs and make practical arrangements to meet them, rather than to engage with them to promote change at a more personal level. Certainly, practitioners at the time often expressed anguish at the loss of more therapeutic functions and what they saw as a waste of the full range of their skills and knowledge (Rachman, 1997). It is ironic that the moment of professionalisation for social work with older people has become so closely associated with a sense of de-professionalisation among social workers, since gerontological social work is an area rich in complexity and potential for emancipatory practice (Ray and Phillips, 2012).

Hospital social workers' involvement with children declined over the course of the 1990s, although this was not only the result of the increased volume of discharge planning work. Anxieties brought about by high profile service failings related to child protection had led to the re-emergence of specialised social work teams during the decade (Payne, 2005), with the result that child protection duties were concentrated in community teams, and hospital social work, aside from a few specialist posts usually funded by charities for specific childhood medical conditions (which are not the subject of this book), was tasked with focusing only on adults. The withdrawal of hospital social workers towards care planning for elderly patients meant that duties such as pregnancy termination assessments were gradually withdrawn from the hospital social worker's remit.

Underlying the NHS and Community Care Act 1990, and the system of social care that has evolved from it, was the ideology of consumer choice and the rule of the market. The tradition of social work as relational casework performed by a benevolent and knowledgeable expert had been under a sustained critique from both sides of the political spectrum throughout the 1970s and 1980s. From the left, social work was criticised as a form of policing aimed at sustaining the interests of capital (Brake and Bailey, 1975), while, from the right, the altruism of all would-be professions was called into question, as were the academic and evidential credentials of social work itself (e.g. Brewer and Lait, 1980). The emphasis on the citizen as a consumer of services who could make choices (Griffiths Report, 1988) was therefore a challenge to the perceived paternalism of social work as a would-be profession. It was argued that ending the state's monopoly on service provision would give rise to services that were more flexible and based on the needs of citizens, rather than of the producers of services. This approach is potentially harmonious with the aims of the disabled people's movement, which suggests that people should be regarded as experts in their own lives and should be enabled to assume control of their own situation wherever possible (Campbell and Oliver, 1996). For the social workers performing this function, their professional role would be less about applying expert knowledge to a passive recipient, and more about using inter-personal skills and practical knowledge to promote individuals' empowerment and connect them to the appropriate resources. Alongside the rhetoric of empowered consumer choice, however, the community care reforms also placed an emphasis on limiting state spending, meaning that the social work role has become heavily associated with determining eligibility for services and gatekeeping resources (Lymbery and Postle, 2015).

The need to maximise limited financial resources in the provision of social care has been accompanied by a widespread reliance on managerial techniques to monitor and direct the performance of workers, in an approach commonly known as 'new public management' (Clarke and Newman, 1997). Managerial techniques tend to emphasise outcomes that can be measured quantitatively, with an emphasis on tangible and calculable activities (Ritzer, 1996). It has been argued, however, that the quantitative measures that are used by social work managers as key performance indicators reflect the priorities of the agency rather than the users of services (Harris, 2003). Critics of the manage-rialist approach argue that it leads social work away from its roots in a holistic understanding of individuals towards the execution of technocratic compe-tencies in the mode of disengaged bureaucrats (Dominelli and Hoogvelt, 1996). Concerns are widespread among social workers that social work is at risk of de-professionalisation, since the therapeutic skills that used to be drawn on are no longer required (Ellis et al., 1999). The success of new public management in dominating social work is reflected in the greater policy influence of the Asso-ciation of Directors of Social Services over that of BASW (Payne, 2005).

With the rise of managerialism, emphasis has been placed on the technical rational components of practice, in which actions are broken down into a system of routines and procedures (Fish and Coles, 2000). The rise in con-sumer consciousness and consumer activism has led those who use expert knowledge in their work to focus increasingly on the management of risk (Beck et al. 1994). This is particularly true of practices in which there is potential for reputational damage (Power, 2004) and can lead to defensive ways of working, focusing on justifiability and auditability, to the detriment of adaptation to specific circumstances (Horlick-Jones, 2004). This has led to an increased reliance on standardised assessment tools and an emphasis on audit culture, often at the expense of human interaction (Rogowski, 2010). As will be explored in Chapter 5, with particular reference to Bauman's (1989) cri-tique of bureaucracies, the dehumanising effects of managerialist culture have been felt particularly in hospital social work, where it is demanded (and has even been legislated for) that social workers produce their assessments quickly and facilitate discharges with minimal delays.

It may be instructive to compare the technical-rational care management approach that has come to dominate contemporary hospital social work in the UK with the more holistic approach that continues to underpin social work practice in adult mental health services. Like the almoners, psychiatric social workers founded a professional association fairly early in the development of their occupation, in 1929, and pursued a distinct professional identity until merging with BASW in the 1970s (Sackville, 1988a; Sackville, 1988b). Social workers in the field of mental health have not seen their work become dominated by the neoliberal care management model to the same extent as hospital social workers, and continue to carry out a role that incorporates therapeutic and emancipatory work, focusing on social inclusion and recovery, with statutory roles related to resource allocation and the detainment of people for treatment of mental health conditions (Allen, 2014). Payne (2005) argues that the Mental Health Act 1983's confirmation of the role of the social worker as a defender of mental health patients' legal rights and counter-balance to medical opinion, through the formal Approved Social Worker role, afforded mental health social workers protection of their specialised role. While the Mental Health Act 2007 opened up the role of Approved Mental Health Professional (AMHP) to other members of the multi-disciplinary team, thus weakening social work's unique status in this area, social workers continue to lead the AMHP workforce (Allen, 2014). By contrast, the Mental Capacity Act 2005, which has particular relevance for social workers who are concerned with older people, allows any professional to make a mental capacity assessment or to be appointed as a best interests assessor. The apparent de-professionalisation of community care social work may therefore be seen to derive from the legislative context that allows only for social workers to act as brokers of care and has not afforded the protection for a more holistic approach as seen in the case of mental health social work.

The benefits of the care management system to the users of services have been equivocal because the reforms were driven not only by a desire to improve the lot of the citizen in receipt of services, but also to cut state spending (Lymbery, 2001). This has resulted in practice that is often orientated around preserving budgets, rather than providing meaningful choice to individuals about the services that they can have (Lymbery and Postle, 2015). Emphasis on identifying the most pressing need means that lesser, yet still significant, levels of need can be overlooked, and expectations of services lowered (Tanner, 2013). A further criticism made of the marketisation of social care is that the users of services do not have the power or freedom to exercise real consumer choice, since the state still purchases care on their behalf, often through block contracts and service-level agreements (Dustin, 2007). Thus, care management is not driven either by the choices of the users of services or by genuine accommodation of their needs, but by consideration of budgetary constraints and best value (Gorman and Postle, 2003). In a context of rising need from an ageing population (ONS, 2015) and constant pressure on financial resources (Lymbery and Postle, 2015), however, it is difficult to refute the necessity of measures to ensure that limited resources are deployed as effectively as possible. For hospital social workers, this often results in the obligation to address the dilemma of either prioritising the need of the individual in front of them, no matter the pressures of competing demands for services, or actively assisting an overstretched system on which so many others rely, at the expense of pursuing the best possible result for that one individual. Legitimate questions can be asked as to the justification for the current limitation of resources, but social workers' employment by the state restricts their ability to engage in political activism as part of their professional practice.

Conclusion

Care management continues to be the dominant model for hospital social work in the UK, and the next chapter will consider recent refinements to this approach, alongside other developments in hospital social work around the world. For now, it is worth drawing some conclusions from this narrative account of hospital social work's history.

The early almoners set out on a project to develop a new professional practice, which aimed at alleviating the social causes of ill health and promoting understanding of the impact of poverty and deprivation on people's health. Achieving recognition as a profession was a struggle for the early pioneers of the occupation, perhaps because of the uncertain and cross-disciplinary nature of their knowledge base and almost certainly because their practitioners were predominantly women, in a highly patriarchal society. The success of almoners and medical social workers in eventually achieving a degree of professional recognition is testament to their ingenuity, determination and assiduousness. It also suggests that their work's value came to be recognised by their medical colleagues. While the hospital social workers of today perform a vital function, undertaking complex, potentially liberating work, often in extremely challenging circumstances, the scope of their role is far narrower than was envisaged or intended as the profession emerged. The narrowing of the scope of the hospital social work role is due largely to the effects of the NHS and Community Care Act 1990 and the decision of the government of the time to restyle adults' social workers as care managers, which should be understood within the wider context of liquid modernity, as discussed in Chapter 1. This demonstrates the powerful effect that coming into the employment of local authorities has had. The fact that social workers are in the employment of the state, to carry out statutory duties, means that they are unable to obtain the professional power to define how they work and lack influence in the shaping and direction of legislation and policy.

Social administration has always been part of social work's role, yet the history of hospital social work reminds us that there is potential for social workers to fulfil therapeutic and liberating functions as well. If there is any desire within the profession to reclaim these former roles beyond the statutory functions of present times, then social workers may need to seek to be employed outside of local authority departments. If hospital social workers had remained in the employment of the NHS, it is doubtful that their role could have been changed so radically, so quickly and easily, since it was valued by clinicians. The wider range of hospital social work practice did not disappear because social workers were not wanted inside hospitals – indeed, the fieldwork for the later chapters of this book found that clinicians repeatedly expressed the wish for more presence from social workers. There is still potential for people with social work knowledge and skills to perform valuable interventions and meet myriad unmet needs beyond the limited (yet vital) remit of discharge planning. To fulfil this potential, hospital social workers will need to find ways of redefining the scope and limits of their practice – and be prepared to fight again for recognition.

Note

1 In cases where agencies other than local authorities (e.g. charities) provide funding for social work posts in hospitals, social workers of course may have a different remit. These are few in number, however.

3 The current state of hospital social work

Introduction

This chapter examines the state of contemporary hospital social work both within the UK and further afield. While there are national and local variations in the policies and practices of medical settings, hospitals in the developed world conform to a homogenous bio-medical model, in which the expertise of the doctor, with support from nurses and other professionals, is brought to bear on the physical illness of the patient (Waddington, 2011). This is not to say that hospitals are not influenced by the cultural setting in which they are placed, or that regional interpretations of biomedicine do not vary considerably. Generally, however, hospitals' institutional cultures around the world are based on a broadly uniform hierarchy of knowledge and authority, in which the roles and expectations of each professional discipline are roughly similar (Bradby, 2009). For this reason, research on practices within hospitals from one country is often transferable to the context of another country, as long as variations of culture, prevailing ideology and custom are understood and acknowledged.

Practices range from country to country and, while discharge planning is consistently a key task, in many countries hospital social workers have a wider range of roles than in the UK. A recurring theme throughout international examples of hospital social work is the continuing and ever-renewing relevance of social work to the issues encountered by hospitals and their patients and families. Innovations from a wide and varying range of national contexts demonstrate the potential of social workers to contribute to health care – both by providing direct support to patients and carers, and by contributing a holistic understanding of the patient to multi-disciplinary teams. At a time in the UK when the NHS appears to be lurching from crisis to crisis, with demand constantly ahead of the availability of resources, it is all too easy to imagine that anything other than discharge planning would represent a profligate use of what little time hospital social workers have. Examples from around the world, however, demonstrate that there is real potential for social work to contribute to the development of more sustainable forms of health care. There is some evidence to suggest that investment in social work can provide considerable long-term savings on the cost of health care provision.

The roles of contemporary social workers in hospitals

The UK

Hospital social work is not usually treated as a specialism within the UK – hospital social workers do much the same job as community-based practitioners, they are just expected to do it at great speed. Indeed, some local authorities no longer base any social workers within hospitals in their districts, and even where there are hospital social work teams, community-based social workers often carry out discharge planning if they are already involved with the patient in question. As was noted in the previous chapter, the care management approach has come to dominate hospital social work practice. When this approach was introduced, the balance of power remained with the social worker both as the 'expert' assessor and as the gatekeeper of resources. The rise in market ideology, however, in which citizens are understood as 'consumers' of services, coupled with increasing self-advocacy by service user movements, has led to a critique of this approach in favour of empowerment of individuals through their direct involvement in the planning and management of their own care (Lishman et al., 2018). Recent social policy developments throughout much of the UK have sought to transfer the choice over which service provider to contract to the users of services, through direct payments and personal budget schemes. These enable individuals to choose their own care provider and negotiate aspects of their care, and to pay them from a personal budget provided by the local authority (Gardner, 2011). The process, labelled 'personalisation' (Leadbetter, 2004), requires that social workers assess the needs and eligibility of individuals to receive a personal budget and review the provision on a periodic basis, while the individuals choose and manage the service they employ.

Lymbery and Postle (2010) have observed that personalisation further limits social workers' already reduced opportunities to engage in therapeutic or emancipatory forms of practice. While this may be the case, there is nonetheless crucial relationship-based work for social workers to do in advising and assisting individuals during the planning of their services, and therefore there are still opportunities to use skills and knowledge in ways that go beyond a purely administrative function (Gardner, 2011). What is most powerful in reducing the opportunities for social workers to undertake therapeutic or emancipatory work is not the transfer of power over service selection to individuals, but rather the intrinsic requirement of the care management system that a tangible outcome, in the form of an eligibility assessment or care plan, must always be the result of any social work intervention. This is especially true for hospital social work, where focus is so strongly on the discharge of the patient.

Personalisation can provide a greater sense of control over their lives to the people who rely on care services in the long term, and has been experienced as particularly empowering by adults of working age with physical or sensory disabilities and by parents of disabled children (Glendinning et al., 2008). For older people, whose physical health and mental acuity are often declining, however, a personal budget can represent a heavy administrative burden rather than a form of empowerment (Hasler, 2006). Indeed, fear of the administrative burden of managing a personal budget may be a factor in deterring older people from taking up social care services, since numbers of older people using social care services overall are declining (Humphries, 2011). It is especially problematic for hospital social workers to set up personal budgets for older people during discharge planning, not only because of the pressure upon them to accomplish each discharge quickly, but also because of the emotional and social difficulties that are so often present during an older person's stay in hospital. Older people are more likely to turn to social workers for support with managing their personal budgets than any other group (Carr and Robbins, 2009), and good social work practice in setting up a personal budget requires taking the time to understand the individual's circumstances fully and to support them and their family in procuring the most appropriate service. The context of a busy hospital ward, in which an occupied bed is badly needed for a waiting patient, for a patient whose needs and family circumstances are complex, limits the ability of hospital social workers to undertake such work.

Personalisation is a key policy driver in England (Department of Health, 2008), Scotland (Eccles and Taylor, 2018) and Northern Ireland (Gray, 2013). The underlying ideology of consumer choice and market competition has been of less prominence in Welsh social policy, however, with the result that the Welsh government has not followed the rest of the UK in its enthusiasm for personal budgets. Wales places more reliance on inspection and regulatory bodies to promote quality in social care services, rather than competition, and aims to maintain the principle of universal services (Drakeford, 2005). For this reason, social worker-led care planning remains more prominent in social work with older people in Wales. Nonetheless, the Social Services and Well-being (Wales) Act 2014 places the desired outcomes of individuals and carers at the heart of assessment and continues to support the availability of direct payments as an option for those who require care. Central to the Welsh approach is the 'what matters conversation', in which social workers must seek to establish the priorities and desired outcomes of the service user (Welsh Government, 2015). The success of the social worker's intervention is then to be assessed against the goals identified, rather than the objective performance indicators identified by service managers that have come to be the norm. In contrast to the centrality of the individual's choices in personalisation, the Welsh approach aims at co-production of care plans, through close co-operation between the social worker, service user and other relevant parties. Emphasis is placed on drawing on and enhancing avenues of support available through family members and community, with the provision of funded care made available only when all other options have been exhausted. Cynics might note that this system is clearly oriented towards saving money by finding low cost/no cost solutions for people's social and care needs. Nonetheless, the renewed emphasis on the relational aspects of the social work assessment offers an opportunity for social workers in Wales to develop new forms of critical practice with older people. For Welsh hospital social workers, the 'what matters conversation' and the prioritisation of the service user's desired outcomes can strengthen their positioning as patients' advocates. The pressure to arrange swift discharges, however, must limit their ability to engage in assessment of the patient's family and community support systems as deeply as they might wish (Tanner et al., 2015; McLaughlin, 2016).

There appears to be little scope at present for UK hospital social workers to make any other contribution to the care of the growing population of older people than to carry on with discharge planning in the face of urgent need. In many other countries, however, the hospital social work role is more varied, and the contribution of social workers to health care is more extensive. The UK could learn much about the potential of social workers to contribute to more sustainable long-term approaches for managing the rising numbers of older people in need of social care. I now turn to an exploration of some of the roles hospital social workers have in other parts of the world.

Around the world

In suggesting that hospital social workers' roles are more varied in other countries than in the UK, I do not mean to suggest that discharge planning is not still of high importance in their work. By its very nature, all social work is concerned, to some extent, with the wider social context in which an individual exists, and social work's aim is usually to bring about some manner of change in the interaction between that individual and their social world (Davies, 1994). All social work practice conducted inside a hospital therefore must be concerned with the patient's life outside the hospital. Thinking about the patient's life immediately after they leave hospital is an intrinsic part of the work of hospital social workers, however much or little they are involved in making formal arrangements for post-discharge support. The difference between the UK context and other parts of the world is the extent to which discharge planning involves working with the patient and/or their family members on how they behave following discharge, and the range of techniques they employ for this purpose.

The USA provides some instructive examples of the way social workers can employ a holistic approach to discharge planning. The extension of Medicare under the Obama administration brought about increasing concern over high levels of readmission of patients within thirty days of discharge (Barber et al., 2015; Bronstein et al., 2015). This resulted in the initiation of a range of pilot schemes aimed at improving patients' transitions from hospital to community, in which social work has featured extensively. Alvarez et al. (2016), for example, report on a 'Bridge Model', in which Hospital social workers work with inpatients to address psychosocial issues that may lead to readmission, and similar schemes are reported by Barber et al. (2015) and Bronstein et al. (2015). In each programme, the intervention of hospital social workers has gone beyond care planning to incorporate therapeutic techniques such as cognitive behavioural therapy and motivational interviewing to bring about behaviour change in patients. Some of this work (e.g. Bronstein et al., 2015) has also involved community follow-up, suggesting a level of continuity of care not seen in UK hospital social work, where the individual's case is usually passed on quickly to a community team for review following discharge.

One institution in the USA, Mt Sinai Hospital, New York, has been particularly active in investigating the potential of social work to contribute to improving outcomes for older people following their discharge from hospital. One of their innovations has been to reintroduce the social work presence in emergency departments, within their specialist geriatric emergency care units. Alongside planning for community-based care and making links with outside agencies, the social workers are called upon to provide counselling, crisis intervention and liaison with family members (Hamilton et al., 2015). The same hospital has also placed social workers at the forefront of their 'Preventable Admissions Care Team' (PACT) (Basso Lipani et al., 2015). The ethos of the team is to provide support for patient transitions into the community, treating the patient's transition as a series of stages, rather than as a single moment of change from one setting to another. Within this approach, social workers are responsible for assessing risks for readmission and helping to solve problems, which involves coaching patients in health-related behaviours and helping to address psychosocial barriers to compliance with medical plans. Within both schemes, hospital social workers remain concerned with what happens to the patient after discharge, but the scope of their work incorporates therapeutic or pedagogic work directly with patients in addition to making suitable arrangements for community-based support.

Appraisals of the American pilot schemes (see e.g. Alvarez et al., 2016; Barber et al., 2015; Boutwell et al., 2016; Owens and Garbe, 2015) have generally suggested that they do have a positive effect in reducing readmissions within thirty days of discharge. Similar studies in Australia have also shown promise. Simpson et al. (2016), for example, reported on a project in which hospital-based social workers were introduced to provide support to patients and families following a traumatic brain injury, utilising an approach that combines care planning with counselling and education. The social workers in this scheme retained their involvement in making practical arrangements for community care, but also had considerable involvement in helping patients and families to adjust psychologically to the injury and its aftermath. The role of hospital social workers to provide therapeutic interventions around coping with illness is generally well supported in Australia, although some social workers are finding increasingly that their work involves negotiating and providing advocacy on behalf of patients, both with family members and other agencies (Cleak and Turczynski, 2014). Nonetheless, Australia appears to embrace a vision of hospital social work in which direct therapeutic work with the patient is valued. Indeed, there have even been schemes to introduce assistant social workers within hospitals, to whom social workers can delegate the more routine care planning and administration tasks, in order to free up their time for the complex and therapeutic work they see as their 'core business' (O'Malia et al., 2014).

Hospital social work is, of course, an occupation not confined to the English-speaking world and is associated with direct therapeutic care of patients in many different national contexts. In Saudi Arabia, for example, where social work is a fairly recent development, hospital social workers are expected to engage with patients' psychosocial issues using relational and counselling skills (Albrithen and Yalli, 2015). Similarly, social workers have well established roles in oncology in both Sweden (Isaksson et al., 2017) and Germany (Kowalski et al., 2015). These roles encompass both the practical, administrative work around planning for the patient's care outside the hospital and helping the patient and family members to cope with the emotional impact of the disease, its implications and its treatment. The willingness of hospital social workers in so many parts of the world to lay claim to therapeutic roles demonstrates how social work can vary depending on the policy context in which it operates. This reminds us again that, if social work is to maintain a role in health care, it must find ways to influence the social and health policy agendas.

The wide range of roles undertaken by hospital social workers suggests that their range of skills and knowledge must be equally broad. It is worth considering in more detail the skills and knowledge that hospital social workers cultivate and employ.

Skills and knowledge

The roles performed by social workers in hospitals around the world require not only the ability to assess people and make plans for their safe care after hospital, but also to engage them directly in work to address their feelings about their health and their health-related behaviours. Programmes to address readmission rates in the USA, for example, draw upon therapeutic theories and techniques including motivational interviewing, cognitive behavioural therapy, crisis intervention and systemic theory (Hamilton et al., 2015; Boutwell et al., 2016; Basso Lipani et al., 2015). In North America, where bachelor-level and masters-level qualifications command differential levels of pay and are associated with differential degrees of expected competency (Salsberg et al., 2018; Grant and Toh, 2017), many hospital social work jobs require the higher Master of Social Work (MSW) qualification, and formal recognition as a licensed clinical social worker for social workers in hospital settings in the USA is available only for those who hold the MSW (National Association of Social Workers, 2017). This demonstrates recognition that the social work role in hospitals is specialised and requires a high degree of knowledge and skill.

Social workers in Canada who hold the lower bachelor's degree are still able to practise in hospitals, but are allocated tasks seen as less complex, such as discharge planning and resource advice (Grant and Toh, 2017). It is ironic that discharge planning is perceived to be a less complex role for hospital social workers, since it requires skilled interactions with people and can involve helping people to navigate through painful and frightening life transitions

(Tennier, 1997). Bringing about a successful discharge will often require that a social worker performs advocacy, crisis intervention, family systems work and inter-professional liaison (Davis et al., 2004). Even in the UK, where discharge planning is less associated with opportunities to perform therapeutic functions, discharge planning is complex series of steps demanding finely honed interpersonal skills and a holistic perspective that draws on ecological systems theory (Heenan and Birrell, 2018). The breadth of skills required is highly taxing for practitioners, who must negotiate high levels of personal politics and respond flexibly to the demands of both patients and colleagues (Pockett, 2002). Often it is impossible to accomplish a patient's discharge without being involved in conflict resolution and family mediation (Sims-Gold et al., 2015). Indeed, although the task of discharge planning has a fairly tangible outcome, since services are identified and provided for the patient if they are deemed in need and eligible, hospital social workers recognise the importance of the nature of their interactions with patients, and tend to evaluate their own work in terms of processes and patient satisfaction, rather than concrete results (Shapiro et al., 2009).

While social workers in hospitals can claim to perform therapeutic functions even when carrying out tasks that appear predominantly administrative, a recurring challenge for any therapeutic work is that it tends to be time-limited by the length of the patient's stay in hospital, which is outside the power of social workers. Indeed, it is not unusual for hospital social workers to have only one contact with an individual. In Australia, for example, Gibbons and Plath (2012) estimated that such work accounts for around 10 per cent of the workload. Hospital social workers tend to see single session interventions with patients as less legitimate than longer term work, despite the obvious range of skills required to carry out such work in a satisfactory way (Gibbons and Plath, 2006). Single contacts between hospital social workers and patients require sensitive handling and may involve intensive work to help patients through a period of crisis. Gibbons and Plath (2012) found that single session hospital social work contacts often follow a complex process through which the social worker must help with some aspect of managing the immediate situation, provide an explanation of the hospital system, help the patient to identify goals, provide practical assistance, negotiation with other professionals or advocacy, signpost for other relevant services, and provide an effective closure that does not leave the patient feeling confused or rejected. Repeatedly meeting such needs requires an extraordinary amount of knowledge, skill and resilience.

The broad range of skills and high levels of personal resilience often demonstrated by hospital social workers make them able to respond with impressive adaptability to unusual crisis situations. The involvement of social workers in Singapore and Canada when dealing with the SARS crises provides an example of this. Social workers in a paediatric unit in Canada were called upon both to help families to manage their emotional response to the crisis and to negotiate between families and various levels of hospital management (Gearing et al., 2007). Similarly, social workers in Singapore set up telephone lines to provide both educational and emotional support to those affected by SARS and their families, drawing on a wide range of theories and skills to help them to cope with the demands of the situation (Rowlands, 2007). That hospital social workers in such widely different cultural settings proved so capable of coping with this crisis is evidence of high levels of professional competence.

Although the adaptability and resilience shown by hospital social workers are admirable traits suggestive of well-developed expertise, the broad utility of social work within the hospital setting can result in social workers being cast as general 'fixers' who can be called upon to bring their problem-solving skills to bear on any type of problem. In Canada, Craig and Muskat (2013) found that hospital social workers identified several roles they play within their work: 'Bouncers', when dealing with challenging behaviour by patients or relatives; 'Janitors', when carrying out tasks no other professional is prepared to do (e.g. finding a dead patient's relatives); 'Glue', when resolving conflicts and supporting patients, families and staff; 'Brokers', when facilitating communication and negotiation between patients, families and doctors; 'Fire fighters', when providing crisis intervention; 'Challengers', when providing advocacy for patients, and 'Jugglers', when swapping quickly between these various roles. Being adaptable and pragmatic is one of social work's strengths, but the applicability of social work knowledge and skills to so many different human issues can mean that it is difficult for social workers to specify what is and is not their role, unless they have very clear guidelines. This means that, within the context of a busy hospital in which clinicians tend to try to avoid work outside their specialism (Latimer, 2000), social workers can easily find themselves called upon to do work that members of other occupational groups do not want to do.

If the skills and knowledge of hospital social workers are to be appreciated properly, in the current era of evidence-based medicine and financial discipline, hospital social work must be able to make some demonstration of its efficacy. This can be difficult, since the outcomes towards which social workers aim are often defined by the individual and may be difficult to quantify. Further, there is a tendency among social workers to give knowledge gained through empirical research less priority than theoretical insight and personal experience compared to other hospital-based occupational groups (McDermott et al., 2017). Data are often collected, but may not be used to demonstrate productivity, with the result that the value of social work within the hospital setting is not made easily visible (Kossman et al., 2006). Social work in for-profit hospitals generates no revenue itself and its ability to contribute to the efficient running of a hospital is not easily proven (Rizzo and Abrams, 2000). It is surprising, in view of the prominence of evidence-based practice in hospitals, that hospital social work has not produced more research aimed at examining its efficacy.

Some studies that have attempted to demonstrate the usefulness of social work within the hospital setting have found that there is little evidence that social work makes an immediate, quantifiable impact within the hospital itself. Kitchen and Brook (2005) examined a pilot scheme in a children's hospital in Kansas City, in which social workers were nominated as the central co-ordinator for each child's care, meaning that all patients were assessed by a social worker. While medical and nursing staff reported satisfaction with the results, such as problems being identified earlier, increased comprehensiveness of care and more orderly discharge, quantifiable effects such as length of stay and bed turnaround were not affected. Similarly, Auerbach et al. (2007) found that the patients referred to social workers had significantly longer stays in hospital than those who did not see a social worker during their admission. Rather than suggesting that this is evidence against the effectiveness of social work in hospitals, however, they argue that this is evidence that social work is most required where patients have complex needs requiring a multi-profes- sional approach. Rizzo (2006) found that there was a link between stroke patients having lower overall medical bills and high levels of informational support from social workers, but otherwise found that stroke patients who were given low levels of social work support tended to use rehabilitation services more effectively. Again, the targeting of social work at the most disadvantaged patients makes its contribution to efficiency difficult to prove.

If the positive impact of social work inside the hospital has been difficult to demonstrate, the recent social work-led schemes in the USA to address read- mission rates provide a welcome suggestion that social work can make a demonstrable contribution to improving health care. Basso Lipani et al. (2015) found that the PACT programme at Mt Sinai Hospital, New York, reduced readmissions at thirty days by 34 per cent, at sixty days by 22 per cent and at ninety days by 19 per cent. The cost saving of the improvement in the thirty-day readmissions in that one hospital alone was approximately $900 000. The Bridge model produced a similar reduction by 30 per cent in thirty- day readmissions (Alvarez et al., 2016). These are significant findings, not only because they demonstrate that social work in hospitals can justify its presence through financial savings, but more importantly they measure what social work in hospitals sets out to do, which is to improve the health chances of the patient after they have left hospital. Lowering a patient's chance of being readmitted is a demonstration that hospital social work can help people to gain the fullest benefit possible. This has been the aim of social work in hospitals from the very early stages of its development.

Being able to demonstrate efficacy in some way is vital to the standing of social work in hospitals. Generating and using research in hospital social work will be discussed further in the next chapter. The final section of this chapter will now explore some of the challenges social workers face when negotiating their place among the various occupational groups contained within the hospital.

Social work's status in hospitals

Hospital social work's central task, discharge planning, can be a difficult practice due to issues of staffing capacity within social care organisations, poor efficiency of communication within hospitals and misunderstandings between agencies (Glasby et al., 2004). A key challenge for social workers is that they must work within a number of different systems both inside and outside the hospital (Jackson et al., 2001). Hospital social workers' ability to act as a link between different services, and between the hospital and the patient is often highly valued by nursing and medical staff (Bywaters et al., 2002). The linking role can be challenging for hospital social workers, since they often must negotiate with multiple institutional logics and span their work across multiple organisational boundaries (Harslof et al., 2017). Time pressure on hospital social workers is compounded by the growing emphasis on shortening inpatient stays and the increasing complexity of patients' needs for post-hospital care (Kennedy Chapin et al., 2014). Additionally, there often appears to be a deficit in the capacity of social care services, meaning that patients stay in hospital for longer than their medical need requires, causing frustration and tension between social workers and health care professionals (Mann, 2016).

Despite its justifiable claims to therapeutic functions, a recurring theme throughout the history of hospital social work has been the struggle for recognition of social workers' expertise and professionalism within the hierarchy of hospital professions. Beddoe (2011) argues that social work is a 'guest' within hospital settings, in that social work's person-centred, strengths-based approach tends to challenge the dichotomy of patient and expert professional. Though there may be contribution to managing the patient's emotional state during an inpatient stay, the social worker's role is to address the needs of the individual in the context of their social environment, rather than to assist in curing a diseased body. This is a nebulous task, and hospital social workers' claim to a discrete body of knowledge seems weak compared to those of clinicians. Just as social work's claim to professional knowledge appears comparatively weak within the hospital, social workers are less able to make displays of professionalism through the ongoing cultivation of expertise and participation in research. Compared to other occupational groups within the hospital, social workers are given little time or resources for personal and professional development (Judd and Sheffield, 2010).

A common concern expressed by social workers in multidisciplinary settings is that they feel that their work is poorly understood by other professionals. Tellingly, Abramson and Mizrahi (1996) found, when carrying out a study on physicians' and social workers' views of inter-professional cooperation, that hospital social workers were much more likely to evaluate the collaboration in terms of how far they felt respected by their medical colleague, whereas the physicians were more concerned with the perceived competence of the social worker and how much they were kept informed about progress. The social workers' interest in the respect of physicians is a reflection both of the power held by physicians and of the tenuousness of social work's professional status. A further source of frustration for hospital social workers with regard to their standing within hospital hierarchies is that their work often relies on collaboration with other professionals, whereas clinicians are often able to carry on work within their own specialisms without relying on others (Albrithen and Yalli, 2016; Craig et al., 2015). This means that social workers' expertise is often obscured by the fact that their achievements are brought about through a team, rather than solo, effort.

The lowly status of social work in hospitals is particularly problematic for practitioners because of their need to influence the decision-making of doctors and nurses (Nelson, 2000). While not a task unique to social work, advocacy has a long-established place in social work practice (Sosin and Caulum, 1983) and social workers within hospitals often find themselves in the position of challenging the recommendations of clinicians on behalf of patients. Professional standing is therefore not merely a matter of self-esteem, since social workers need a sense of authority in order to be able to advocate effectively. Similarly, where hospital social workers act as a link between hospital staff and the patient and carers, it becomes vital that the social work role is understood and respected. Effective discharge planning relies upon social workers' ability to maintain co-operative working relationships with other professionals (Glasby, 2003). Where hospital social workers' professional prestige is diminished, their ability to act on behalf of patients is similarly diminished. The professional standing of hospital social workers is therefore not merely a matter of practitioner self-interest, but of concern in their ability to provide the best possible service for patients and carers.

A claim that hospital social workers make across all countries is that their input offers a holistic approach to patient care, which can enhance the lived experiences of patients and their family members. Hospital social workers argue that they move beyond their clinical colleagues' medicalised focus on functional deficits and bodily disease to engage with the wider context of individuals' lives and the social and structural issues that impact on their health (Craig et al., 2015). While hospital social work's claim to offer a uniquely holistic approach within the hospital team might be contested by clinicians who do pay attention to the bio-psychosocial model of disease (Barry and Yuill, 2016), social work does have the quality of being an occupation whose usual location of operation is within the community, rather than the hospital. It therefore comes naturally to social workers to focus on the social functioning of patients and to incorporate the role of informal carers in their understanding of an individual's world (Nilsson et al., 2013). Many clinicians therefore recognise the added value social workers bring to hospital teams in understanding the social dimensions of patients' lives.

While hospital social workers often welcome the increasing interest of clinicians in the psychosocial aspects of health care, some are beginning to perceive a threat to their role from other professional groups' encroachment on their roles. The role of social workers in discharge planning can come under pressure due to resource constraints, with the result that other professionals are sometimes called upon to do the work of social workers (Judd and Sheffield, 2010). Further, Chan (2014), while exploring the contribution of social workers to palliative care in Hong Kong, notes that the uniqueness of social work's value base is under threat from nurses and physicians as they attempt to develop a more holistic approach to their clinical work. Isaksson et al. (2017) note a similar threat to Swedish oncology social workers from their nursing colleagues, a problem exacerbated by social workers' lack of systematic training in the psychotherapeutic approaches on which social workers are expected to draw. Indeed, the authors note that a third of the social workers in their study had undertaken additional training in psychotherapy, suggesting that the knowledge base of social work within hospital settings may not stand up to scrutiny for some of the roles to which social workers might lay claim. The tasks that social workers have the unique knowledge and skills to perform are valued within hospitals, but if social work does not articulate and continue to develop its unique and eclectic knowledge and skill base, these tasks may be taken over by other occupational groups.

Conclusion

Hospital admissions often mark a transition in a person's life, as they move from a time of better health to a time of disability, long-term illness or even terminal decline. Social work has the potential to assist people through this time of transition, both by engaging in work to support the individual's emotional and psychological coping, and by intervening in the wider social systems upon which that individual may rely. In many parts of the world, hospital social workers undertake a mixture of practical, administrative, emancipatory and therapeutic tasks in support of hospital patients. Discharge planning remains a prominent task for hospital social workers throughout the world, of course. This reflects the fact that social work is orientated to see the individual within their wider social context. Social work's critical stance towards power structures and oppression means that practitioners sometimes pose a challenge to the authority of clinicians and take on the role of the patient's advocate. In order to be an effective support for patients, both in terms of their adjustment to the circumstances of their illness, and in terms of the workings of power relations and structures upon them, social workers need to carry a certain amount of professional authority within hospitals. Achieving such authority is a continuing struggle for social work, both because of uncertainty over its knowledge base and because of the difficulty in proving its efficacy. Recent studies in the USA have indicated that hospital social work can be effective in reducing readmission rates within 30 to 90 days of discharge. This offers considerable savings in terms of health care costs and, more importantly, improves the lived experiences of those who are assisted to gain the greatest possible benefit from their medical treatment.

In the UK, much of the potential of hospital social work is going unused. Local authority employment within the care management system means that UK hospital social workers' practice revolves around the swift and efficient arrangement of social care, so that patients who do not need further inpatient care can be discharged as soon as possible. Developments in the care management system that focus on individuals' choices strengthen hospital social workers' role as advocates, but the mechanism of personal budgeting is difficult to set up under high pressure to discharge patients who are often still weak and vulnerable. The discharge planning work for hospital social workers is not going to go away, but an expansion of the presence of social workers in hospital could bring substantial savings to the NHS by lowering readmission rates, and improve life for many people who struggle to cope with the physical, mental, emotional and social implications of living into advanced old age. This would require a wider remit for social workers, to provide direct therapeutic work and to become more actively involved in managing patients' transitions from hospital to home. Establishing such a role for social workers requires long-term vision and willingness to invest in preventative approaches to social care.

4 Using research in social work

Introduction

This book is concerned both with what hospital social work is now, and what it could be. If we are to consider developing the role of social work in hospitals, and in health care more broadly, then we need to give careful thought to how we understand the basis of our knowledge claims and the evidence upon which we draw in support of our practices. Thinking about social work's knowledge base is no less the responsibility of individual practitioners than it is of managers, agency directors, policy-makers and academics. At stake is our understanding of what it means to be a good, professional social worker. Is good social work simply the fastidious implementation of government policy and legislation by culturally sensitive officials who observe a code of practice that protects their integrity and impartiality, or can it also be a critical practice drawing on empirical and theoretical knowledges, derived perhaps from multiple disciplines and sources, but organised into a coherent understanding of its methods, values and purposes? This chapter seeks to outline an approach to using research evidence in social work that will enhance social workers' capacity to use research to enhance the criticality of their practice. Much of the discussion will be of general relevance to social work, but I frame my approach with particular reference to hospital social work.

Evidence-based practice

In the present day, it is impossible to discuss social work's relationship with research without giving at least a nod to the evidence-based practice movement. The origins of evidence-based practice are in the field of medicine, in which systematic reviews of randomised control trials first began to challenge common practices (Sheldon and MacDonald, 2008). An oft-quoted definition of evidence-based practice is that it is 'the conscientious, explicit and judicious use of current best evidence in making decisions about the care of individuals' (Sackett et al., 1996, p. 71). The original model of evidence-based medicine suggests a hierarchy of evidence upon which physicians should draw when making decisions about a patient's care. At the top of the hierarchy sit systematic reviews of randomised control trials, followed by single randomised control trials, then cohort studies, case control studies and single case studies (Oxford Centre for Evidence-based Medicine, 2011). By using whatever such evidence is available, combined with clinical experience and the preferences of the patient, the physician is then able to decide the best course of action for treating the patient's disease (Sackett et al., 1996).

Evidence-based medicine rose to prominence because of its potential to make clinical practice safer, more consistent and more cost-effective, through grounding medical practices in scientific, empirical evidence rather than investing authority in the judgements of senior physicians purely on the basis of their length of experience (Greenhalgh et al., 2014). The attractions of the evidence-based practice model for social work are twofold: it offers professional authority to the occupation through the identification and development of a discrete body of expert knowledge, and it offers a moral basis for social work interventions. The development of knowledge about social work is problematic, as will be discussed further below, but it is worth first exploring the moral arguments in favour of an evidence-based approach to practice, so that we can be clear if this is something worth attempting, however fraught with difficulties it may prove to be.

Proponents of evidence-based practice argue that it is an ethically sound way of approaching any public service, since it shares with people who use services the fruits of rational enquiry and ensures that flaws in practice founded on consensus, anecdotal evidence or tradition can be exposed and replaced by practices more likely to be successful (Sheldon, 2001). For Gambrill (2001, p. 172), this places the responsibility for engaging with research evidence on individual practitioners, since their efforts to help others can be accused of being 'insincere' if they are not 'caring enough' to find and appraise research findings related to their field of practice. In other words, the need for an evidence base for practice arises from the personal responsibility that social workers take when they become involved in the lives of others. As Marsh and Fisher (2005) note, the decisions that social workers make can have a significant effect on people's immediate circumstances and may be of great influence in shaping their futures. Morally, therefore, social workers need to be as informed as they can be about the likely and potential effects of the decisions they make and the actions they take. Chalmers (2003) argues that research evidence should be used to adjudicate what the best practice or course of action may be, suggesting that practices can be prescribed based on the best available evidence. Advocates of evidence-based practice do acknowledge, however, that the values and preferences of individual people must also be an integral part of the decision-making process and, where the evidence is not clear enough to point unambiguously to one course of action, allow that the practitioner's own personal experience should be drawn upon (Sackett et al., 2000). The values and perspectives of the person using services are vital considerations because even the most widely efficacious interventions may not be suited to every individual.

Evidence-based practice appears to satisfy the criteria of ethical practice according to the three main ethical paradigms through which our conduct can be considered: deontology, teleology and virtue ethics (Banks, 2012). From a deontological perspective (i.e. a perspective that argues that we have a duty to do things that are right, and to avoid doing things that are wrong, regardless of the consequences), the principle that social workers must seek out and follow the best way to help people would be difficult to contradict. From a teleological perspective (i.e. one that focuses on the consequences of actions as criteria for understanding their moral worth), evidence-based practice is satisfactory because it focuses on the outcomes of social work interventions. When we carry out practice based on evidence of the efficacy of our chosen approach, we do so in the hope of achieving the best possible consequence for the people with whom we are working. (This does not mean, of course, that we should consider the ends to justify the means with any type of social work practice. If an intervention is abusive or oppressive – for example frightening people into complying with medication regimes – the fact that hospital admissions may be reduced does not excuse the practitioner's actions.) Finally, the 'conscientious, explicit' use of evidence (Sackett et al., 1996, p. 71) also satisfies a post-modern conception of ethical practice as involving self-examination and the will not to deceive (Foucault, 1984) – and therefore provides a justification of evidence-based practice within the framework of virtue ethics. From a Marxist or Feminist perspective, however, social work interventions that focus only on the individual may be argued to serve only to promote small improvements in circumstances without challenging the oppressive social structures that produce disadvantage in the first place (Jordan, 1990). Such an objection can be countered by pointing out that improving individual circumstances is often emancipatory and challenging of social structures (Thompson, 2016) and, further, by considering that improvement in an individual's circumstances ought to be recognised as something desirable, whatever structural or systemic injustices remain.

What's wrong with 'what works'?

The strength of the moral case for the evidence-based practice movement naturally leads to the conclusion that we should seek evidence about the successes and failures of our interventions in social work, and base our practices upon that evidence. In other words, that we should seek to establish what works, and do that. The problem for social work is that establishing what works is far less straightforward than is the case for medicine. When we attempt to build practice based on evidence generated through the social sciences, a range of philosophical and practical difficulties with the nature of knowledge assail us. Ultimately, these must not deter us from using evidence to inform our practices, but they do prevent us from simply transferring the model of evidence-based medicine into social work unaltered. We cannot treat the knowledge derived from social science research in the same way that medicine treats knowledge produced by the natural sciences.

A key objection to a purist transfer of evidence-based practice into social work is that it is based on a naïve, positivistic conception of epistemology, in which it is assumed that the social world is understandable through objective, value-free analysis (Du Toit, 2012). However, social research can rarely, if ever, be separated from the subjective experience and values of the researcher (Denzin and Lincoln, 2011), meaning that it is difficult to identify research that can claim to reflect the realities of the world objectively. Postmodernist theory suggests that social realities are constructed by the effects of language, which reflect power structures and enable some representations of reality to dominate over others (Rossiter, 2000). Any scientific claims of knowledge about the social world are therefore seen as contentious, since we cannot know the social world outside the constructs and power relations provided by language. This is of crucial importance to social workers, since their work generally involves attempting to provide assistance to people who are in the grip of power, rather than people who wield power (Dominelli, 2004). It is all too easy for social research to replicate the power structures of the society in which it occurs, perpetuating disadvantage and oppression. Research evidence, therefore, cannot simply be trusted by social workers – they must be able to examine it critically and consider its positionality in relation to power and social structures. This certainly does not mean that research evidence regarding outcomes and efficacy of interventions is unusable, but it makes it more complex to produce research evidence that can be used for this purpose.

Just as our ability to know the social world objectively is highly contested, the methods by which we gain evidence about the social world are far from clear-cut. The evidence-based practice movement favours randomised controlled trials and systematic reviews of randomised controlled trials, yet these can rarely be produced without methodological objections in social research. Significantly, it is not possible to have a 'blind' control group, because people who use a service are always aware of whether or not they are receiving an intervention (Hammersley, 2005) – there is no placebo. Further, the practices of those delivering interventions cannot be standardised because they involve human behaviour, which is unpredictable and multi-faceted. Both practitioners delivering interventions and people receiving services may respond in myriad ways to circumstances and conditions that cannot be controlled or accommodated within the research design. Practice settings often vary greatly from research settings, meaning that interventions can rarely be replicated in everyday practice as they are performed during research trials (Witkin, 2017) and practitioners themselves are unpredictable and inconsistent in how they carry out social work interventions (Webb, 2001). In summary, the evidence-based practice movement's emphasis on practitioners replicating what has been seen to work elsewhere rests on the fallacious assumption that human behaviour is predictable and that social work interventions can have a predictably determining effect on the future choices of free human agents, whose circumstances and motivations are almost infinitely complex. There is an important distinction between knowing that a particular intervention *can* be successful and knowing how, where and when to employ it (Witkin, 2017) and this latter knowledge is not readily available from research reports.

An important practical objection to the evidence-based practice movement is that the emphasis on measuring outcomes naturally requires collection of data, but the process of collecting and reacting to data comes to have a restrictive influence on practice (Geyer, 2012). The need to provide information about outcomes is frequently fulfilled by gathering quantitative data, which can then be fed into audit systems which rely on targets and performance indicators as a means of managing performance (Power, 1997). Such an audit culture can work well when data collection is easy and when the policy choices are clear cut, but is less likely to work in areas where causality is difficult to establish and where all the structures at work are not clearly visible (Geyer, 2012). Unless audit systems are able to take account of all the complexities of a given situation, they are likely to induce a see-saw effect between policy responses for supposed crises and supposed successes, since they often make the flawed assumption that if performance is improving it will continue to improve, or vice versa (Geyer, 2012).

In addition to the epistemological and practical problems with a purist evidence-based practice approach, the influence of Marxist and Feminist theories in social work means that it would never be enough for social workers to know simply 'what works'. 'What works' must be understood within the context of social structures which can be oppressive to those without power in society (Dominelli, 2002). Thus, social workers need to ask whether 'what works' is working in favour of an oppressive social structure or in favour of the oppressed. Social work's engagement with issues of structural oppression is central to its identity (Millar, 2008), meaning that narrative evidence of the realities of service users' social worlds will always be significant to practitioners. We must therefore think very carefully about asking the right questions. If we take the case of hospital social work, as was noted in the previous chapter, there is emerging evidence from the USA that social work interventions in hospitals can reduce the number and frequency of readmissions of patients within thirty and sixty days (Basso Lipani et al., 2015; Alvarez, 2016). While this suggests a welcome reduction in physical injuries or health complications for people, we do not know whether those patients simply return to lives of loneliness and isolation, or have other ongoing social issues that may not result in the need for hospital care, but nonetheless impact on their overall well-being. If hospital social workers focus only on health issues and overlook patients' wider social systems, the gains made by their interventions will be limited.

Critical best practice: the middle path

So far, I have identified a moral case for evidence-based practice and a list of practical and philosophical problematisations of outcome-based research knowledge as a guide for social work practice. The issue is not an intractable one, however, and is amenable to a sensible, middle-path approach. Ferguson (2003b; 2008) has described a model of 'critical best practice', which is envisaged as a process through which social workers can integrate identification of methods of intervention that have been seen through rigorous research to be helpful with the use of critical theory as an interpretive framework for understanding the wider social structures impacting on individuals' lives and engaging with the values of people who use services. This allows the social worker not only to be able to appraise and utilise empirical research on practical interventions, but also to seek to develop and draw upon insight into the social worlds of people who use their services, and the wider structural influences affecting them. A critical best-practice approach satisfies the moral claims of evidence-based practice by enabling social workers to draw on appropriate research evidence in planning and developing their practices, while providing enough flexibility for social workers to incorporate a critical understanding of the workings of power within people's lives. Research evidence is used as part of a decision-making process, rather than as a narrow command that certain methods of intervention must be undertaken (Gray et al., 2013; Plath, 2014). This approach acknowledges the place of discerningly selected research-based knowledge in practice, but also gives weight to the values of both practitioners and people who use services, and to the practice wisdom of experienced social workers.

The role of practice wisdom is somewhat overlooked in the purist conception of evidence-based practice, yet there is an intrinsic element of artistry in social work, through which specialised knowledge is blended with intuitive skill and tacit knowledge. Social workers require more than knowledge that can be transferred through instruction, whether written or in the classroom, and more than instrumental knowledge about how to follow procedures or employ techniques. Good social work practice also calls for *wisdom* about how to respond to particular situations, circumstances and contexts (Petersén and Olsson, 2015). There are times when social workers must challenge conventional understandings of social phenomena and question standard responses to the needs with which people present to services. In the case of hospital social work as currently practised in the UK, the task for the social worker with almost every patient is to facilitate their discharge as soon as possible. For many patients, this will be the right thing to do, but for some individuals, for example those who are subject to abuse within their families or whose homes are hazardous in some way, a more measured and investigative approach is required. Uncovering abuse or poor care often requires close attention to people's verbal and non-verbal presentation that may not be consciously understood by the practitioner, who may instead describe a 'gut feeling'. Similarly, social workers' communication with people using their services requires an intuitive ability to improvise and respond in the moment to individuals. A critical best- practice approach should not fetishise such practice wisdom to the point of claiming that it trumps all other forms of knowledge, but recognises its place alongside research evidence in making decisions about how to proceed in practice.

While the critical best practice approach enables us to strike a compromise in how we adapt evidence-based practice for social work, there is also a need for flexibility in our understanding of what counts as acceptable evidence. The hierarchy of evidence within evidence-based medicine risks devaluing important forms of research in social work and exaggerates the significance of evidence based on the paradigm of natural sciences (Petersén and Olsson, 2015). Whilst knowledge based on randomised controlled trials can be useful in informing social workers about the potential effects of certain intervention approaches, there are other forms of research that can be equally useful to social workers, through informing critical reflection and self-awareness in social workers, and raising consciousness of the perspectives of people who use services. Being accountable in their practice means not only that social workers should seek to carry out interventions that seem likely to benefit people, but also that they should undertake practice that takes due care of people's dignity and human rights, that challenges oppression and that values people and their strengths (Witkin, 1996; Witkin, 2017). This means that social workers need to engage with a wide range of types of research evidence without privileging any one type over another, certainly incorporating quantitative and qualitative methods, but also articulating the full range of human experience through valuing equally the voices of those who are marginalised.

In addition to empirical research, it is important that social workers continue to take interest in developments of theory related to sociology, social policy and psychology, since these are crucial in underpinning and renewing the value base of social work (Ferguson, 2008). Social work values must not be considered to be static and settled, but should be dynamic and open to question. Drawing critically on theories of how people and societies work is necessary since theorisation, in the form of assumptions about the nature of people and society, is inevitably part of social work practice (Thompson, 2010). Engagement with social theory, in particular, is also vital in guiding social work research and informing social workers' appraisal of empirical research. Social work must use theory to enhance reflection and to examine honestly its underpinning values and assumptions, but also must use research to examine and develop the theories underpinning practice.

Incorporating research in critical best practice

Empirical research for social work can be divided into three main subject categories: research about people who use services; research about social workers' and social work organisations' practices; and research about the impact of social work interventions on the lives of people with whom they are carried out. All three subject categories are of equal importance in critical best practice, because they all inform different elements of the processes through which social workers make decisions and think about their work. Crucially, none of these forms of research should be expected to dictate how social workers practice. Instead, they should be seen to help social workers to make informed judgements and decisions, and to assist them in the process of reflecting on their practice.

Research about people who use services may be derived from a wide range of disciplines and may conform to a wide range of ontological and epistemological paradigms. Just as it is necessary for social work to resist a hierarchy of evidence that privileges research which mimics the positivistic approach of the natural sciences, it is also important to avoid a form of 'inverse snobbery' in which such research is said to be of no value. To take the example of knowledge related to health, whether mental or physical, empirical research is constantly produced from a wide range of disciplines including biomedicine, nursing and other allied health professions, sociology and psychology. Government agencies may commission this type of research, but it may also be produced by non-governmental organisations and self-advocacy groups. All of these can be avenues of knowledge for social work. The importance of this type of research to social work is that it gives us some knowledge about the nature of population groups who may be in need of our services. Before we even think about our approaches to working with people, we have to know something about their circumstances and the types of need with which they may present. Social workers are likely to be able to understand and interpret their face-to-face encounters with people more accurately if they are able to contextualise them within a wider understanding of the conditions and workings of the society in which those people live their lives. If we think back to the early days of social work, the Charity Organisation Society initiated case work based on the belief that much of poverty was self-inflicted, and without an understanding of the social structures that lead to widespread and unavoidable deprivation (Payne, 2005). The research work of Seebohm Rowntree (1901; 1918) in the UK was vital in providing social workers with an account of poverty that was based on empirical findings rather than assumptions and prejudice, enabling social work to begin to develop an understanding of the role of social structures and power in the creation of human problems. In the contemporary era, huge numbers of both quantitative and qualitative studies about the lives people live are available and social workers need to be aware of the messages that come from them to help them to appreciate the developments and trends of the society and culture in which their practice is located.

An important caveat must be heeded by social workers when drawing on cross-disciplinary research about people who use services: the more the research evidence points towards justifying social work in taking actions that restrict the freedoms of individuals and families, the more critically the evidence must be appraised. For example, Wastell and White (2012) have observed how claims from neuroscience regarding the irreversibility of damage to the infant brain have led to a 'now-or-never' approach to the protection of infants thought to be at risk in their parents' care, yet they suggest that the evidence that chaotic or neglectful parenting can cause permanent damage to the brain is weak. Social workers do not appear to be actively engaged in critically analysing this evidence, and yet it is allowed to drive their practices (Plafky, 2016). The emerging study of epigenetics is starting to make similarly bold claims to those of neuroscience, that may lead, for example, to a disproportionate focus on the behaviours of mothers during pregnancy and their child's early infancy (Wastell and White, 2017). These must be critically analysed by social work if they are to be allowed to influence social work practices. Social work must not allow itself to be 'blinded by science' when it comes to the claims of medically orientated research but must apply the same 'respectful uncertainty' to scientific claims as is required in the investigation of abuse. This is an especially important trait for hospital social workers to maintain as they work in an environment in which the claims of medical science are routinely taken for granted.

While social work can and should draw on research findings derived from other disciplines, it is also necessary to pay heed to research that explores social work practice explicitly. This type of research aims to explore the nature of social work organisations and social work practices, to consider the extent to which we treat people justly and, indeed, whether we as practitioners are treated justly within the organisations and systems in which we work. This form of research holds up a mirror to social work, to help social workers to appraise their positionality in terms of power relations with people who use services and within organisational structures. The purpose of such research is not to tell social workers how to do their work, but rather to raise consciousness and deepen reflection on practice. It is to this genre of research that the empirical findings of this book (found in Chapters 5, 6 and 7) belong. The aim of these chapters is to bring to light the ways that bureaucratic systems direct and constrain practice in contemporary social work practice, to explore the values that are enacted by social workers within these systems and to highlight the particular challenges social workers face working within hospitals as institutions. It is my hope that these chapters will raise social workers' awareness of the power and resilience of their values and will help them to question and challenge the excesses of bureaucratic restrictions imposed on them by the organisations that employ them.

For the purposes of deepening reflective practice in social work, which is very much at the heart of the critical best practice approach, ethnographic research (upon which the subsequent chapters of this book are based) is particularly helpful. Ethnography in social work research has been used extensively to explore the organisational and institutional cultures of social work and the way social workers generate and share practice knowledge (e.g. Pithouse, 1987; De Montigny, 1995; Scourfield, 2003; Helm, 2016). While such studies tend to feature data gathering almost exclusively within the social work office (Ferguson, 2016), there is an emerging body of work using mobile methods to uncover the practices of social workers during direct contact with the people to whom they are providing a service (e.g. Longhofer and Floersch, 2012; Holland et al., 2011). Ethnography is particularly suited to social work because it facilitates theorising the particular-in-context (Floersch et al., 2014), enabling social workers to explore the application of theory to practice as it is constructed in the everyday world. Helpfully for hospital social work, ethnography also has a long-established pedigree in medical

settings, which has brought to light the ways through which medical behaviour and knowledge are transmitted and perpetuated within clinical settings
(e.g. Becker, 1961; Atkinson, 1995; Latimer, 2000).

The third and final genre of research for social work I have identified,
research regarding the impact of social work practice on people's lives, is the
genre in which the evaluations of outcomes and efficacy so beloved of the evidence-based practice movement belong. Appraising outcomes and judging the
success or failures of social work interventions is not the only purpose for
research of this genre, however. Research studies of this kind can also give a
voice to the people who receive social work services, providing insight into how
social work practices are received and helping social workers to understand
how their positionality with regards to power and social structures looks and
feels from the point of view of people they seek to help. If the correct questions
are asked, they can also help us to understand the impact of social work practices beyond the simplistic performance indicators and outcome measures
often used as proxy measures for social work's success or failures. For example,
it is often the responsibility of social workers to arrange packages of home care
for older people who are in need of additional support to continue living in
their own homes. A simplistic evaluation of social workers' success might
incorporate measures such as how long the person receiving such a care package managed to continue living without suffering further accidents or dete-
rioration in their abilities, or how satisfied they were with the social worker's
efforts on their behalf, or even how quickly the social worker managed to make
the necessary arrangements. A more critical approach to considering the
impact of the social worker's practice, however, might seek to understand the
overall impact of the setting up of the package of care on the person's well-
being. Callaghan and Towers (2014) found substantial evidence to suggest that
older people who live in residential care or extra care housing feel more in
control of their daily life than people who receive care at home. Remaining at
home is often a preferred option for older people who need care (Windle et al.,
2009), but the best outcome for them may be to leave their home in favour of a
more communal form of housing and care provision. Social workers who are
aware of research evidence in this regard will be better placed to have informed
conversations with older people about their best interests, and may be more
able and inclined to help them to consider a wider range of care options.

Embedding research in practice

Social workers who wish to draw on research evidence to inform their practice
need to go through a process of identifying relevant research, appraising critically the strength of the evidence and then deciding the extent to which the
answers offered are applicable to the real-life situation with which they are confronted (Morago, 2006). This implies a level of engagement with research that is
unfortunately rare at present among social work practitioners outside those
actively engaged in social work education, whether for qualifying or post-

qualifying awards. Social workers' use of research evidence in making decisions about their practice is low and inconsistent (Sheldon et al., 2005; Bellamy et al., 2006). Many social workers do not actively engage in reading and appraising research on a regular basis, but tend to rely on dissemination of research findings through training and continuing professional development events in which research-based knowledge is presented in easily digested formats (Plafky, 2016). Research cannot be embedded into social work practice unless ways can be found to assist and encourage social workers to become more actively involved in accessing and reading research findings critically.

As Walter et al. (2004) point out, direct engagement with research by practitioners is not the only way in which social work can use research. Research can be embedded into policies and guidelines at national and local levels or can be promoted by leaders within organisations. Mosson et al. (2017) found that social work managers do consider keeping up with research evidence to be an important part of their role but are not systematic in searching for and using research evidence. Even where legislation, policy, guidelines and procedures for social workers have their roots in research evidence, the extent to which research can influence the practices of social workers who do not engage directly with research evidence will be limited by social workers' independence in their day-to-day work. The core work of social workers frequently takes place in people's homes, away from the oversight of policy-makers and managers, making the world of individual social work practice a private one (Pithouse, 1987). For this reason, the concept of the 'street level bureaucrat' (Lipsky, 1980) remains relevant to social workers, since social workers retain the discretion to interpret policies and to use them in idiosyncratic ways (Evans and Harris, 2004).

At present there is a deficit in the organisation of social work inasmuch as research and practice appear to be two distinct and loosely connected fields of practice. The looseness of the connection is not helped, of course, by the limited access social workers have to academic journals, which is only slightly and inconsistently alleviated by the emergence of open access publication. There are also formidable barriers to social workers' engagement with research, caused by their working conditions. In the current economic climate, social work departments are expected to carry out ever increasing amounts of work with fewer staff and time for individual social workers to examine research and reflect on its implications for practice is, therefore, extremely scarce. Reading research is rarely seen as something that is a legitimate use of working time and the pressure of conforming with targets measured by performance indicators means that many social work employers simply do not value the curiosity and knowledge-seeking in social workers which are vital if a working culture of research-based practice is to be fostered (Newman et al., 2005).

For the use of research evidence to become a more integrated part of everyday social work practice, the working culture of social work teams needs to change. Skills and knowledge about research methods learned during qualifying courses can quickly be forgotten and newly qualified social workers can easily be assimilated into a working culture that bases its practices on authority, tradition and preference rather than clear evidence of the most effective interventions (Sheldon and MacDonald, 2008). A potential challenge to this might be made by the creation of posts of practitioner-researchers within social work teams. A practitioner-researcher might either spend a part of every working week carrying out research, or perhaps more practically, might take a period of weeks or months as sabbatical time, to carry out a piece of work related to that team or agency's aims. Alternatively, just as academics can be 'bought out' of teaching and administrative duties when awarded a grant for a research project, practitioners with the necessary competency could be 'bought out' to contribute to projects. The skills employed by social workers in practice and researchers overlap so closely that some have even suggested that they amount to the same task (McNamee and Hosking, 2012). There is great potential, then, for practitioner research not only to improve the quality of social work practice, but also to enhance the quality of research.

A key benefit of the creation of practitioner-researchers within social work teams is that it would keep discussion of research current within social work teams, both during formal meetings and informal discussions between colleagues. Further, periods of sabbatical to undertake research might aid retention of experienced staff by giving practitioners a break from the highly stressful 'coal face' of social work practice, which causes many social workers to leave the profession (Van Heugten, 2011). The role of a practitioner-researcher also has potential benefits in terms of the research evidence it is possible to produce. Having knowledge of the workings of an agency means that practitioner-researchers may have an advantage in working out how to capture and analyse their data and, crucially, in ensuring that the research findings are put to use in making a difference to agency policy, management and practice (Robson, 1993). Of course, the role of practitioner-researcher does not come without attendant difficulties as well. The pressure of work within social work teams may mean that practitioner-researchers are put under pressure to neglect their research in favour of casework. Further, they are likely to need guidance in planning and carrying out their research, which may have cost implications. For researchers investigating a world with which they are intimately acquainted, there is also the problem of making the familiar strange, so that they are able to say something new about the area they are studying (Delamont and Atkinson, 1995).

The proposal to create social work practitioner-researchers is intended to address the problem of the lack of familiarity with, and use of, research evidence within local authority social work teams. The creation of such practitioner-researchers would not only create a new and potentially fruitful source of research data for managers and policy-makers but would also introduce a much-needed culture of referring to, discussing and evaluating research within social work teams. The potential benefit of creating such a culture outweighs the difficulties and added costs which might be associated. Piloting the role of the practitioner-researcher could be of particular benefit in hospital social work, if the potential of social workers to provide expand their roles in health care (as discussed in the previous chapter) is to be realised. Hospitals are institutions in which the conduct of research is not only normal but even expected and therefore the role of practitioner- researcher within hospital social work may advance the standing of social work among clinicians and help social work to strengthen its claim to an expanded role in supporting people with health-related social needs.

Conclusion

In this chapter I have attempted to set out how social workers can balance practice-based expertise, social work values and empirical evidence about social work. There is no need to regard these three components of social work knowledge as competing – all are essential if social work is to realise its ambition and potential as a source of assistance and adjuvant to empowerment for people. The current division between social work practice and social work research is disadvantageous to both sides, where no 'sides' are needed at all, resulting too often in research that does not ask the right questions or provide meaningful suggestions for practice and impedes the ability of social workers to identify and use helpful research to inform their practice. If the status quo is to change, then the barriers need to be broken down between researchers and practitioners. Good research can inform social workers about the needs of population groups, can guide practitioners towards helpful and effective working methods and can inform deeper reflection. The creation of practitioner-researchers, whether as permanent parts of local authority social work teams, or through 'buying out' social workers' time, offers the possibility of breaking the stale and unproductive status quo and enabling social work to find innovative ways of meeting the evolving challenges of life in the contemporary era. Social workers need to be less willing to be told what to do by policy-makers, organisations and managers and more able to think deeply about the direction of their practice. Engaging with research critically is essential to this endeavour.

Part II

An ethnographic account of hospital social work

Preface

Chapters 5 to 7 present findings from an ethnographic study of a hospital social work team. I was interested in the nature of the tasks hospital social workers (HSWs) perform and how HSWs perform them, the extent of managerial and bureaucratic control over their activity, the extent and nature of HSWs' discretion, the nature of relationships between HSWs and other hospital professionals, the nature of HSWs' relationships with patients and carers, and the ideologies and moral principles that underpin HSWs' decision-making. Such interests appeared to call from the outset for 'thick description' of HSWs' activities as witnessed through participant observation (Geertz, 1973), to be supplemented by interviews and analysis of HSWs' written outputs. My aim was to understand the social world in which hospital social work is performed from the perspectives of those who co-create this world – meaning not only the HSWs, but also patients, carers and members of staff within the hospital who have direct dealings with HSWs.

In setting out to produce any qualitative research, the researcher should be clear about the ontological and epistemological assumptions underpinning her/his work. I reject the 'naïve' positivist notion (Denzin and Lincoln, 2011) that it would possible for me as an ethnographic researcher to access an objective 'real world' unspoiled by my observation of it. Instead, I assume that the social world and our knowledge of it are constructed by the actors within it (Berger and Luckmann, 1967), meaning that reality will vary for each actor depending on her/his personal history and status within the historical and cultural context. Some (e.g. Hennink et al., 2011; Lecompte and Schensul, 1999) have argued that acceptance that there can be plural versions of reality leads to a position of absolute relativism, in which it is impossible to make any claims of truth since any assertion could be declared equally valid as any other. I reject such a position, and instead rely on Hammersley's (1992) 'subtle realism'. That is to say, I assert that there is a world that carries on whether it is observed or not but accept that my knowledge of this real world can never be complete, whatever method is used to study it. Ultimately, my fieldnotes, however imperfect, and the theories and interpretations that arise from them, are based on events that happened.

I carried out my research fieldwork within a typical large general hospital in an urban area of the UK. This involved participant observation and informal conversations over a total of 30 working days spread over a number of months, supplemented by in-depth interviews with participants. The social work team focused almost exclusively on discharge planning for patients in advanced old age, many of whom presented with issues regarding their mental capacity to make their own decisions regarding future living arrangements. The team consisted of eight social workers, two senior practitioners, a manager and two administrators. It was sub-divided into a unit responsible for arranging care for those already known to the local authority and a unit responsible for assessing patients for new packages of care, which tended to involve longer-term and more complex work. Additionally, four doctors, four nurse managers, four occupational therapists, two physiotherapists and eight staff nurses were formally engaged as participants, as well as three patients and seven informal carers. This enabled me to access parts of the discharge process in which social workers were not present, such as ward rounds, and permitted some limited observation of social workers' interactions with patients and carers. Where patients or (in the case of patients with mental incapacity) carers had given their consent, I was able to view social workers' case files and analysed these both as factual records of actions taken and as representations of social workers' rhetorical representations of events and actions (Taylor and White, 2000).

I approached analysis of my data according to some of the principles of grounded theory (Glaser and Strauss, 1967), in which theory is inductively produced from the accumulation of evidence. I used coding and memo writing to develop categories from which theories could emerge, while maintaining a constructivist understanding of the nature of my data – i.e. that my data are a constructed product of my interactions with participants and the meanings that we bring to our world (Charmaz and Brynant, 2016). Thus, I reject Glaser and Strauss's (1967) argument that theories are 'discovered' through the data, and instead regard my theoretical insights as constructed through the interactions that constituted my data collection (Charmaz, 2014).

5 Social work in the 'iron cage'

Introduction

This chapter explores the nature of the hospital social work role and the way hospital social workers accomplish their work, examining the tasks they undertake and the systems which organise and control their practices. I argue that the role of the contemporary hospital social worker (HSW) is essentially to fulfil a series of bureaucratic functions related to arranging the care of the patient after discharge. The term 'bureaucratic' is to be understood in the Weberian sense, in which there is a rigid allocation of labour, a hierarchy of authority and regular or continuous execution of assigned tasks by those qualified to perform them (Weber, [1922] 2015). Analysis of the key tasks performed by the HSWs will demonstrate the extent to which the bureaucratic system dehumanises patients and encourages dehumanising practices by HSWs. This is not to suggest that the HSWs observed should be considered officious or unfeeling – indeed, Chapter 6 will examine ways in which they enact humanitarian social work values and demonstrate personal commitment to patients – but rather to highlight how the bureaucratic system in which they work restricts the forms of practice in which HSWs can engage. Despite the restrictions, HSWs retain some discretion in how they approach their work and their use of this discretion – both on behalf of patients and in their own interests – will be explored.

Discussion of the dehumanising influence of the bureaucratic system in which the HSWs practise will draw on the work of Zygmunt Bauman. Bauman (1989) argues that the same social conditions that culminated in the Holocaust are present in the instrumental rationality that is central to all modern bureaucratic systems. Instrumental rationality focuses on finding the most efficient means of achieving a goal, rather than whether the goal itself is acceptable (Weber, [1922] 2015). Bauman suggests that bureaucratic systems enable instrumental rationality by separating the decision-maker from the human impact of their decision, and by separating the implementer of the decision from responsibility for taking it. Such systems therefore discourage their workers from engaging with the moral dimensions of their actions, instead encouraging them to focus on efficiency and compliance. The moral disengagement of bureaucrats is further strengthened by the way in which the bureaucratic system minimises their direct contact with the people whom their actions affect. Several aspects of Bauman's analysis of bureaucracy can be seen in the system within which HSWs operate.

The duties performed by the HSWs on behalf of patients fall into two main categories: designing packages of care (POCs) for patients who are ready for discharge, and taking part with clinicians in the assessment of patients for NHS-funded Continuing Healthcare (CHC), which is allocated to patients with on-going complex medical needs. Striking about both tasks is the extent to which the social workers are concerned with management of the failing body or failing mind, as opposed to the emotional needs of the patient, or their social circumstances beyond their need for daily care. The definition of need in hospital social work is confined to aspects of the patient's bodily or mental functions which are preventing their discharge from hospital, with scant regard to the wider issues of the patient's emotional, psychological or social well-being. This does not mean that the HSW's role becomes entirely mechanistic – often HSWs are called upon to negotiate with family members and carers, for example, or to mediate in complex disputes between family members. Further, establishment of patients' wishes and advocacy for them to achieve the outcomes for which they hope is a central feature of much of the HSWs' practice. Such practices, however, are accomplished with the explicit end goal of patient discharge always in mind.

Managerial control of social work practice

As was noted in Chapters 2 and 3, UK social workers in all community care settings are subject to managerial oversight and 'new public management' techniques designed to increase efficiency and guarantee value for money. For the HSWs, two managerial systems – that of the NHS and that of the local authority – act to direct their practice and demand the accomplishment of their work as quickly as possible. HSWs' encounters with NHS managers are generally limited to the middle managers, chiefly those who are responsible for 'patient flow'. Senior HSWs from both the fast response and long-term sections of the team were observed to have regular meetings with NHS patient flow managers to identify problems with delayed discharges and explain what the social work team is doing. For the fast response senior HSW, this involved a daily meeting with the patient flow manager in a busy office within the hospital.

> The two of them look at a list of patients on a computer screen, which uses colour coding to highlight patients who are considered medically fit for discharge but are waiting for other services before they can leave the hospital. HSW7 gives updates on what is happening where social work is the cause of the delay and the patient flow manager corrects the system where the cause of delay is found to be a service other than social work. There is no space in the computer system for a full explanation – instead,

a drop-down menu is used with categories to pick from that explain the delay – e.g. 'awaiting social work allocation'; 'occupational therapy' etc.

(Fieldnote)

The focus on the computer screen and its colour coding has a dehumanising effect on the construction of the patient, who is reduced to a unit which must be shifted, rather than a person with unique needs and a unique history. Such dehumanisation is a vital component of bureaucracy, helping to separate the completion of bureaucratically required tasks from the moral engagement of the worker (Bauman, 1989). The effect of such dehumanisation within the hospital is to encourage NHS staff and the HSWs to prioritise the efficient discharge of the patient over wider issues of social, emotional, psychological or spiritual need that the patient may present. The focus on efficiency in place of the holistic approaches of HSWs in other countries discussed in Chapter 3 may be misplaced, since those wider personal issues may have a significant impact on bodily and mental functioning.

In the rehabilitation wards, the senior social worker overseeing the longer-term cases had a meeting once a week with the patient flow manager, who would be joined by occupational therapists, a discharge liaison nurse and various ward managers, who came in for an allocated time slot. One of the HSWs summed up the patient flow meeting thus:

It's called patient flow but really I think they mean impatient flow! It's all about chasing people out. You'd like to imagine it's a bunch of people coming together trying to do their best for patients – that's what we'd all like, I suppose. But really it's about people using leverage, trying to get what they want.

(Fieldnote – HSW3)

The HSW here is arguing that attendees of the meeting seek to prioritise tasks that they consider necessary above the best interests of each individual patient. The use of leverage between professionals suggests that the interests of each agency are of more importance than making the right decision for the patient. This suggests that instrumental rationality is an important driver of hospital managers' practices, with efficient work towards an end given priority, and consideration of whether that end is truly desirable remaining of secondary importance.

In addition to the pressure for HSWs to facilitate discharge exerted by NHS managers in person, sometimes the wards take direct action to apply pressure. On one occasion, a HSW highlighted to the team manager a number of referrals to the team for patients who were not yet fit for discharge, and a number of patients who were referred to the team but discharged by the ward before they had been seen by a social worker. The team manager commented,

That's health's way of stomping their feet when we have a waiting list.

(Fieldnote)

The nature of the team's role means that there are always patients waiting to be seen, but if the bed flow managers perceive an unusual delay, they sometimes adopt the approach of discharging patients who require a social work assessment unseen by social workers in response. For ward staff, the moral claim of the patient whose medical needs no longer justify a hospital bed, yet who could not return home safely, is in competition with the moral claim of the next patient whose medical need is now greater. The impression given to social workers is that of a system in which they must immediately serve the needs of patients as they are presented, or accept that the patient will return to the community without the care that should be provided. This is recognised by the HSWs as a deliberate strategy to induce speedier discharge work – as real as other, more officially sanctioned forms of pressure. Any moral obligation a HSW feels towards the patient with whom they are currently occupied is therefore in competition with concern for the patient who may be missing out. The effect of this can be seen in one HSW's description of feeling guilty if she spends too much time with one patient:

> [Y]ou partly feel, if you spend a long period of time with someone and you come back to the office, you've got other cases, you partly feel guilty for spending that time.
>
> (Fieldnote – HSW10)

While Bauman (2000b) argues that bureaucratic processes diminish consideration of the moral aspects of social work action by placing focus solely on the efficiency of task accomplishment, this HSW's comment is a reminder that efficiency itself has a moral claim on social workers. There is, after all, an ethical imperative for the distributors of publicly funded services to ensure that such services are provided to appropriate recipients and with minimal waste (Ferlie et al., 1996). HSWs are driven not only by the managerially demanded bureaucratic imperative of efficiency, but also by a sense of obligation to share their resources as fairly as possible. Radical social work theory offers the critique that such practice does not tackle the inequalities underlying the need to ration services (Brake and Bailey, 1975), yet unless social workers work to meet the immediate needs of people who require services by whatever means at their disposal, they are failing them (Ferguson, 2003a).

Where social work is felt to be the cause of too many discharge delays, the patient flow managers will 'escalate'. This means passing on information about the delays to senior NHS managers, who will then contact senior managers within the local authority employing the HSWs to press for a solution. Tellingly, there is little face-to-face contact between the hospital social work team and senior managers from the local authority. Local authorities' senior managers are responsible for the allocation of the resources suggested in HSWs' care plans and for directing social workers in complex situations. However, they are housed in another building in a different part of the city and are rarely, if ever, seen in the hospital. Thus, there is a clear separation between decision-makers and the decision – a separation which Bauman (1989) argues is central to the dehumanisation which enables bureaucracies to pursue efficiency without moral judgement of the end result. This separation is amply illustrated in one HSW's experience of 'escalation'. The HSW, assigned to a patient who was frequently admitted to hospital for apparently fabricated symptoms, was keen to carry out an in-depth assessment in order to find a long-term solution to her frequent presentations, prior to her discharge. Clinical colleagues failed to attend meetings that the HSW called or simply refused to become involved at all, and soon the patient's delayed discharge was 'escalated' by the patient flow manager. Discussions were held between senior managers from the hospital and the local authority (none of whom had direct contact with the patient) and the end result was that the patient was sent home from the hospital without the assessment that the HSW had wanted to do being completed. Removed from the sight of or engagement with a person who is suffering, senior managers are able to make a decision that serves the end of immediate, efficient bed clearance, ignoring the moral claim of a suffering person to real aid (Bauman, 2000b). The result in this case was that the patient was discharged from the hospital and given the same services she was receiving before her admission, and returned as an inpatient within a few weeks. Ironically, the ruthless pursuit of efficiency therefore can produce inefficiency, since the problems this patient presented remained unresolved and would continue to take up clinicians' and HSWs' time on her next admission.

As with all local authority social work teams, the HSWs' performance is appraised by managers and the government department through key performance indicators (Gregory, 2001). For NHS managers within the hospital, the key performance indicator is the length of the patient's stay, and the length of time the patient is waiting for a discharge while considered medically fit. For local authority managers, key performance indicators are the length of time between receipt of referral and allocation of a social worker, and the length of time for a social worker to complete an assessment and submit a care plan. The emphasis of managerial strategy is therefore firmly on the speed with which the HSWs can expedite discharges and, consequently, efficiency must be valued above all other considerations. While, as was noted above, efficiency does have a moral claim for HSWs who are aware that others are waiting for their services, reduction of risk and ensuring a safe discharge remain key real-world consequences of work done well (Payne, 2014). Where performance indicators do not match the aims of social work practice, either the quality of practice falls (Broadhurst et al., 2010; Munro, 2011), or reporting of practice is manipulated to feign compliance (Wastell et al., 2010). There is therefore a constant tension for the HSWs between maintaining the quality of their work and satisfying the demands of managers.

While the purpose of collecting data on performance indicators is to maintain control over practice (Gregory, 2001), their use is incomplete for the hospital social work team, since there is a lack of clarity about whom the data are reported to and how they influence decision-making from senior managers. For example, on a weekly basis, the team manager collects information from all of the HSWs about impediments to their work that they have experienced through the fault of clinicians, yet it is unclear to them what is done with this information. The team manager commented,

> I just collate it [the data] and send it to the civil service. What they do with it, I've no idea.
>
> (Fieldnote – Team Manager)

Similarly, the team undergo a census of information about delayed transfers of care around every six weeks, which involves senior social workers sifting through data to ensure their accuracy. However, once the census data are sent to the relevant government department, nobody in the team is aware of what is done with them. There is no personal stake in the performance data for the HSWs, since they receive neither reward nor censure according to whether the data are considered positive or negative (Payne, 2000). This weakens the claim of the bureaucracy on the hearts and minds of the HSWs. Bauman (1989) argues that bureaucracies encourage their workers to consider only the efficient completion of required tasks, rather than their moral worth. However, without clarity about how their efficient working contributes to the system as a whole, HSWs' loyalties cannot be fully removed from the patients and carers with whom they work. Thus, doing a job well for the HSWs cannot be limited only to doing the work in the efficient manner the bureaucratic system requires.

HSWs experience both local authority and NHS middle managers primarily as sources of pressure to meet externally set standards for the completion of work. The alliance of NHS and local authority managers to direct the social work team towards completing discharges with all possible speed is reflected in the use of externally set performance indicators which measure the time taken to carry out work. The separation of senior managers who make decisions about the resources made available to patients from the HSWs who must communicate such decisions is part of a dehumanising approach to enable the most efficient work possible. Social workers are aware of the moral claim of efficiency in order to distribute scarce resources as fairly as possible, but cannot be brought wholly into the bureaucratic mentality of valuing only efficiency, since they have no personal stake in the performance data or clarity about their contribution to the larger aims of their organisation.

Fordist and Taylorist approaches to social work practice

While the managerial systems are only partially able to secure the HSWs' commitment to efficiency as the primary consideration for their practice, the day-to-day work performed by the HSWs frequently reflects approaches orientated towards the efficient processing of patients' needs. A key aspect of Weber's ([1922] 2015) description of bureaucracy is the repetitive completion of assigned tasks and this can be seen in the way HSWs describe their work:

It's really about performing assessments on behalf of clients. It's a~~l~~
assessing their needs and their wishes, to try and get them out of hos~~p~~
in the safest way possible.

(Interview – HSW4)

No matter who the patient is, the goal is always the same: to discharge the
patient from hospital. If a patient's discharge depends on receiving a service
from the local authority, this must always be accomplished in the same way:
with an assessment and a care plan. Production of the care plan can be further
broken down into a series of routine tasks: to find out from health professionals
the patient's physical needs; to establish, where possible, the patient's wishes for
how they want to live after discharge; to establish what informal carers (family
members, partners etc.) are willing and able to do to support the patient upon
discharge; to establish the patient's financial circumstances; to identify resources the local authority will provide, and finally to produce detailed instructions
to service providers as to how the patient is to be cared for upon their return
home. Similarly, the outcomes available for patients upon the completion of a
HSW's assessment are limited to just a handful of options including permanent
residential care, temporary residential care, intensive home rehabilitation or up
to four daily visits from hired carers. Thus, in the practices of the HSWs, two
central tenets of Fordism can be seen: the standardisation of the end product
(for Ford, cars that were identical; for HSWs, care packages/residential place-
ments with little flexibility) and the breaking down of a complex process into
smaller, repetitive tasks (for Ford, the factory assembly line; for HSWs, the
repetitive use of standardised assessments) (Dustin, 2007). This is not to say
that the work of the HSWs is devoid of complexity, but rather that the complexity they encounter – for example in a patient's relationship with family
members, or issues related to housing – can only be managed through a process
which has strictly limited outcomes.

The Fordist tendency within the HSW team can be seen in their insistence that
bureaucratic processes for managing patients' needs are followed in every case.
One senior HSW commented regarding ward staff's adherence to procedures:

> One problem is that they sometimes try to bypass us, and ring the care
> agency directly, then discharge the patient without telling us. Next thing
> is, we get a call from the patient saying their carer didn't come. But we
> didn't know they were home and it hasn't gone through brokerage to re-
> start their package.

(Fieldnote – HSW7)

Of note here is the emphasis on the bureaucratic process through which a care
plan must be processed in order for a patient to receive services upon leaving
hospital. Even if the patient is to have the same package of care they were
receiving before they came into hospital, they must be assessed by a social
worker, who can then trigger the brokerage team to re-start the care. The

bureaucratic function of the social work team as the gateway to community services cannot be bypassed by clinical staff, despite their impatience with social workers, who are often unable to respond to the patient's needs as quickly as would be desirable.

The community care reforms of the 1990s were noted for their fragmentation of service provision (Dominelli, 1996; Carey, 2015) and a Taylorist approach in which social work is broken down into discrete tasks that can be handled along a line of social work practitioners, rather than a person's needs being treated holistically by one worker (Dustin, 2007). Taylorism originated as an attempt to make factories more efficient by breaking jobs down into small tasks and studying workers' movements in order to minimise wasted time and effort (Giddens and Sutton, 2017). The Taylorist approach is in evidence with the HSWs in the way that their task is considered to be complete as soon as the patient has left the hospital. Review of the care plan is left for a community team to follow up and is not the responsibility of the HSW who originated it. Moreover, even while HSWs are actively working with patients, significant aspects of practice are considered outside their remit. In particular, the identification of abuse or neglect of vulnerable adults is a key responsibility for social workers (Wilson et al., 2011), yet HSWs have limited opportunities to identify issues and must pass the responsibility on to a dedicated Protection of Vulnerable Adults (POVA) team to direct the investigation if any instances of concern come to light. On one occasion, the team manager was observed explaining to the team that an instance of financial abuse had later been discovered against a patient with whom one of the HSWs had worked. The POVA team had expressed concern that an opportunity to identify the abuse at an earlier stage had been missed by the HSW involved. The team manager acknowledged that the conversation that would have brought the matter to light had not been held by the HSW at the time because it did not seem relevant, adding,

> We don't do as thorough assessments due to time constraints, but if you have more time with a patient and can dig deeper, you're expected to.
>
> (Fieldnote – Team Manager)

The time pressure on HSWs means that they need to make sure that their assessment work is proportionate to each patient's presenting need and, therefore, the depth into which assessments go can vary. Patients whose discharge planning needs appear to be straightforward may be provided with a less thorough assessment, meaning that it is possible for issues of hidden abuse not to come to light, especially since those who are suffering from abuse may not be forthcoming. Failures to identify abuse can therefore result from the HSWs' conditions of work, since they are required to keep their assessments focused narrowly on the discharge plan, and only investigate the patient's wider circumstances where it appears relevant to the plan to do so.

The Fordist and Taylorist approaches noted serve the purpose of efficient processing of work, rather than being orientated towards the needs of individuals in receipt of services. This is not to say that the HSWs are completely unable to attend to building a relationship with a patient or a carer, but that the purpose of that relationship will not extend to engagement in more therapeutic work. Social work assessments, with their strict focus on bodily capability, may not reflect the priorities of patients who are facing a change in lifestyle brought about by declining health. The emotional impacts of such changes are not addressed by the HSWs as a routine part of their work. While HSWs demonstrate empathy in their daily interactions with patients and carers, these interactions are focused primarily upon what is physically necessary to discharge the patient from hospital. The efficient accomplishment of the hospital social worker's task therefore relies on the HSW not engaging with all aspects of a patient's life, but focusing only on those aspects of the person's life which can be aided by the options available in social work care plans.

Dehumanisation

As discussed, the nature of the system within which the HSWs work is such that their ability to engage with the full emotional world of patients is restricted. In many instances, my observations and encounters would suggest that the system works to dehumanise patients. Bauman (1989) argues that dehumanising the objects of any bureaucratic process is essential for optimum efficiency. I do not wish to suggest that the practices of the HSWs are uniformly dehumanising to patients or that the HSWs do not show compassion and human concern on a daily basis – Chapter 6 will explore in detail ways through which HSWs promote patients' human rights and act upon humanistic social work values. Of concern here, however, are the routine practices and processes in which HSWs are involved which do have a dehumanising effect that cannot be avoided or completely mitigated.

The opportunity for HSWs to engage with patients' and carers' emotional worlds is somewhat limited by lack of a confidential space with which to talk while a patient is in a hospital bed. Time is also an inhibiting factor, since HSWs do not have the time to build relationships with patients and carers incrementally, but must quickly establish a rapport strong enough for them to be able to raise personal questions and difficult issues related to a patient's declining health and increasing dependency. Similarly, time constraints mean that difficult conversations with carers must often be conducted over the telephone. A fragment of a typical telephone conversation between a social worker and carer, in this case the wife of an elderly patient, ran thus:

> ... Good lord! Look, I'll check out with my manager if that's something they can still provide ... [carer speaking] Have you ever felt that you need more support for yourself? ... [carer speaking] No, no you couldn't do that yourself because it needs two people to hoist him ... [carer speaking] I'm sorry that he's not coming home today ... [carer speaking] Well, I can't say exactly when because I don't want to get your hopes up when I can't – I

can say I will try and get him out as soon as possible ...[carer speaking] I'm sorry that he's not coming home today ... [carer speaking] Now that he's having two carers it may take a bit longer to identify two carers ... [carer speaking] I know he was disappointed and all I could do was apologise ... [carer speaking] He did feel deflated, yes, yes, ... [carer speaking] Oh you've been married 54 years! Gosh what's your secret? ... [carer speaking] [HSW laughs] You're not going to tell me? ...

(Fieldnote – HSW10)

It would be remiss not to acknowledge the tact and skill displayed by the HSW in this extract. Throughout the conversation she spoke with a clear, loud voice that was sympathetic in tone, matching the expressions of genuine empathy on her face. In this case, the patient had been told by ward staff that he was to be discharged the next day, only for this to be overruled by the HSW, who needed to arrange additional care for him at home. Of note is the extent to which the social worker took personal responsibility for the delay in discharge, apologising repeatedly and emphasising that she had also apologised to the patient. Also of interest is the acknowledgement of the disappointment she has caused, juxtaposed with a personal commitment to do her best, without making promises she will be unable to keep. Throughout this exchange the HSW conveyed a great deal of personal warmth, providing a compassionate face to a bureaucratic inconvenience. While it is clear that the HSW did her best to build a rapport, however, the limitations of relying on telephone contact are also apparent. When the carer disclosed that she had been married to the patient for 54 years and the HSW asked her what her secret was, the carer shut the conversation down. In a face-to-face encounter, it is possible that this remark might have led to a deeper conversation that would involve the social worker engaging with the carer's emotional world and an interaction of therapeutic value might have occurred (Trevithick, 2012). Thus, the working methods of the HSWs minimise their ability to make a genuinely human connection with patients and carers.

Time constraints not only limit the depth of HSWs' personal engagement with patients and carers, but can also give rise to circumstances in which HSWs perform bureaucratic functions on behalf of patients without knowing the patient at all. Where a patient is deemed to lack capacity to make decisions due to impaired mental functioning, decisions are taken through a best interests meeting (BIM), which is attended by the clinicians involved with caring for the patient in hospital, the informal carers or family of the patient and a HSW. Sometimes, the HSW's first contact with a patient is initiated by the urgent request of the ward, because a BIM has already been called before a social worker has even been allocated to the patient. A similar situation often arises for meetings concerning Continuing Healthcare (CHC) – a form of care funded and provided through the NHS rather than the local authority. When HSWs attend any meetings in which they are new to the patient, they perform the function of ensuring that procedures are properly followed and that the rights of the patient are properly observed. For example, they may highlight the fact that a BIM meeting has been called when no capacity assessment has been documented or they may point out the need for the hospital to enact the Deprivation of Liberty Safeguards (Ministry of Justice, 2008). The ability of HSWs to perform these functions even for patients they have not met means that it is preferable for them to attend than for the meeting to go ahead without them. However, where the HSW has better knowledge of a patient, s/he is likely to be able to provide a fuller contribution that may reflect better the priorities of the patient. The fact that HSWs are obliged to take part in meetings with limited knowledge of patients suggests that the smooth functioning of the bureaucratic system is sometimes prioritised above consideration for the patient's personhood. This is reinforced by the fact that the patient is often absent from such meetings, due to mental incapacity or physical ill health. The physical separation of the patient from people making decisions makes her/his dehumanisation in the eyes of decision-makers more easily possible (Bauman, 1989).

The desirability of CHC funding (as it is not means-tested), together with the finite availability of financial resources within the NHS (Klein and Maybin, 2012), mean that it is necessary to have a standardised, fair system for CHC distribution. The system for determining eligibility for CHC relies on assessing patients' needs against pre-determined criteria based on the nature and complexity of the care required. Bauman (2000b) argues that any bureaucratic process to categorise human suffering as classifiable 'needs' is dehumanising and that rigid application of rules of eligibility reduces social workers' ability to engage with the moral impact of their actions. In the case of CHC, a patient's eligibility is determined through a meeting in which health professionals, a HSW, carers and (rarely) the patient are gathered to go through a proforma known as the Decision-supporting Tool (DST) to determine if a 'primary health care need' is present. The DST calls for professionals to class needs as low, moderate or high (NHS, 2018a) – converting the lived experiences of the patient into a quantifiable set of data which can be judged dispassionately. The role of the HSW within the DST meeting is to explore the information provided by the clinicians in detail. For example, the HSW might ask the nursing representative whether the patient is able to express any wishes of their own, or how much agitation s/he demonstrates on the ward. Where an agreement cannot be reached between the HSW and health professionals in the meeting, the matter is referred to a panel of senior managers, who are yet further removed from direct contact with the patient. Thus, fair distribution of resources must be delivered through a highly rationalised, dehumanising system to which the HSWs are bound to contribute.

While there is less emphasis on rigid eligibility criteria in the assessments HSWs complete for local authority service provision, the reduction of people to categorised needs is as clear. HSWs' care plans tend to focus strictly on tasks that hired carers must perform for patients and it would normally be impossible from reading a HSW's care plan to obtain any real sense of the personality or personal history of the person at its centre. The instructions given within care plans can be extremely specific to bodily needs, for example:

... empty ileostomy bag
... use hoist to transfer patient into and out of bed and into and out of wheelchair

Needs outside the successful continuing management of the failing body are not considered to be within the realm of the HSW, and are not given consideration, other than through advice to contact voluntary agencies who might provide assistance during the assessment process. The outputs the HSWs produce therefore follow the same dehumanising process as the CHC assessment, in which the living person is only seen in terms of needs which must be instrumentally fulfilled.

Just as the HSWs' assessment and care plan documents are highly rationalised, the process of purchasing a service on behalf of a patient is similarly impersonal. For example, if a HSW decides that a patient will be able to manage at home with a set number of calls from a professional carer each day, s/he must submit the plan for approval by the team manager, to ensure that the presentation of the patient's needs matches the service that is to be provided. Once the plan has been approved, it is passed on to a separate 'brokerage' team, who will make a contract with an agency to fulfil the duties prescribed by the social worker. The brokerage team is not composed of social workers, but administrators whose role is to manage the contracting of an agency. This process enables the local authority to purchase a service according to its own budgetary priorities, which means the quality of the service will often be of secondary importance or even unknown (Coulshed et al., 2006). The rhetoric of purchaser/provider split as enabling choice for people using services (McDonald, 2006) or of personalisation, in which the service user's voice is central (Gardner, 2011) is therefore overlooked in favour of ensuring a rationalised and efficient service.

Dehumanisation of patients is functional within the hospital social work system both to conserve scarce resources through applying strict eligibility criteria for services, and to enable HSWs to complete work as quickly and efficiently as possible. Routine practices for the HSWs frequently encourage dehumanisation of patients since time for personal engagement is limited and the HSWs' ability to obtain services for patients depends on their ability to present them as an assembly of eligible needs. As will become clear in Chapter 6, the dehumanisation of patients is emphatically not the choice of individual HSWs, but to work in the hospital social work system necessarily means, at the very least, using dehumanising processes instrumentally to procure services for patients.

Discretion

This chapter has so far outlined a bureaucratic system that aims to ensure that the HSWs keep efficient and swift discharge of patients as their highest priority. Despite the control of HSWs' practices through managerial techniques and the limitations on the ways in which they can engage with patients and carers, however, the system also relies on HSWs using a certain level of discretion in their daily work. Evans and Harris (2004) argue that Lipsky's (1980) concept of street-level bureaucracy remains relevant in social work, since some discretion is always retained by practitioners whatever rules, regulations or procedures are in place. Lipsky (1980) argues that social policies are formulated not only by governments through legislation, or by senior managers in charge of developing organisational goals and procedures, but also by government workers who have direct contact with the public, as they must interpret those policies and implement them as 'street-level bureaucrats'. Thus, government or management policies are often reinterpreted and distorted by street-level bureaucrats, who exercise high levels of discretion and autonomy, and whose practices evolve to help them to manage their work in their own interests, whether to cope with a high demand for services, to reduce uncertainty and dilemma, or to give preferential treatment to certain types of citizen (e.g. on grounds of acceptable behaviour or some form of prejudice).

The concept of street-level bureaucracy remains relevant to HSWs because their interactions with patients remain unobserved by managers, and because the eligibility criteria for patients to receive services from the local authority do not eliminate discretion. Eligibility criteria and strict definitions of what needs can and cannot be met by social workers reduce the range of choices available to social workers (Ellis et al., 1999), yet HSWs retain power over how information is presented to the managers who must approve their care plans. Knowing the eligibility criteria well means that HSWs are able to present patients' needs in a way that almost guarantees their receiving a service and it is rare for care plans to be rejected. Where managers do refuse approval for a care plan, this is commonly interpreted by the HSW as a sign that more information is needed, rather than that their interpretation of the patient's needs is wrong. In such instances, the social workers will seek further information from their clinician colleagues, rather than give up on the care plan they have suggested.

The discretion of the HSWs extends beyond how they present information about their patients to secure them services. Despite the expectation that they should expedite discharges as quickly as possible for every patient, HSWs do take more time when they are able and feel it is warranted, for example when the patient presents complicated issues:

Like this case I'm working on now, the husband's got Alzheimer's and has EMI [services for the elderly mentally infirm] involved and now she's not mobilising but she was a couple of months ago and something's telling me there's something underlying, but they're saying she's ready to go and it just sometimes happens. But I'm not letting her go home, and then they think we're just delaying things but they don't see that we have to get to the bottom of things.

(Fieldnote – HSW4)

While the HSW is aware that his management of the case will be interpreted as an unwelcome delay, he is prepared to carry on with what he wants to do without concern over the criticism he may receive. It is interesting that he relies heavily upon his intuition, and places more significance upon this than on the information from clinicians who say the patient is ready for discharge. While Lipsky (1980) and Musil et al. (2004) argue that street-level bureaucrats use their discretion to avoid dilemmas and reduce uncertainty, the opposite is true of the HSW's conduct here. It would be easy to take the clinicians' assessment at face value and provide a swift discharge, but instead the HSW decides to embrace uncertainty and investigate issues which may be underlying the patient's loss of mobility. Of course, the delay to the patient's discharge that the HSW can effect will be limited – it is likely that the patient's case will be 'escalated' by patient flow managers if the situation is not quickly resolved. However, the discretion of the social worker to cause some delay while he makes a deeper assessment demonstrates that the bureaucratic system does not have full control of HSW practice.

Discretion is also called upon when HSWs need to improvise in order to maintain the smooth operation of a patient's discharge in the face of unforeseen difficulties. Such activities correspond to what Craig and Muskat (2013) identified as the 'janitor' role for HSWs, as they carry out necessary tasks that no other professional is prepared to do. With surprising regularity, I observed the HSWs chase up actions that would be the responsibility of other professionals, such as ordering equipment, which is the responsibility of nursing staff or occupational therapists (OTs). Similarly, the HSWs often provide liaison with patients' carers and give them information that is the responsibility of another professional to provide. For example, one HSW telephoned a patient's son to explain that the OT was unable to obtain the necessary equipment for the patient's discharge for a few more days. Following the call, she then felt it necessary to check whether the patient himself was aware of the delay and the reasons for it. When asked why she took this on herself, the HSW shrugged and said that, though she thought the OT *should* make the telephone call herself, she probably would not and then she, as the social worker, would 'get the blame' anyway.

> Unfortunately that's always the process. They think the social worker will do everything.
>
> (Fieldnote – HSW9)

The HSWs' willingness to carry out the 'janitor' tasks despite some resentment that they are not necessarily their responsibility reflects their commitment to patient care, but also to ensuring that the bureaucracy works as smoothly as possible. While, as was noted above, commitment to the bureaucracy is qualified rather than absolute, the HSWs recognise the importance of maintaining the smooth function of the system to discharge patients to the extent that they will cover the roles of other professionals where necessary.

Further, taking initiative in the manner described above is a small act of professional freedom: the HSW grasps the opportunity to use her discretion and expertise to manage a situation and ensure that the plan for which she is responsible works as intended.

While HSWs can use discretion in ways that are orientated towards benefitting patients or carers, there are also examples of working practices that appear to exist to protect HSWs' own interests. An important example of this is the team's policy towards mental capacity assessment. Under the Mental Capacity Act 2005, a mental capacity assessment can be carried out by any professional working with a person whose ability to make a decision may be compromised by lack of ability to understand or retain the necessary information. Social workers' training means that they are well placed to undertake capacity assessments and it is common for them to do so in many organisations (Wilson et al., 2011), yet within the HSW team, very few capacity assessments were performed. Instead, there was an informal agreement, instigated by the hospital's managers and clinicians, that physicians would take responsibility for assessing the capacity of inpatients. This agreement had become such a routine part of practice that HSWs had ceased to question it.

> But generally, yeah, we just kind of push it over to the doctors to carry out capacity assessments, and I don't really know why, because it would make sense if we're doing it when we're most involved.
>
> (Interview – HSW9)

Despite explicit encouragement from their team manager to become more involved with assessing mental capacity during one team meeting that was observed, the HSWs did not change their practices during the fieldwork. When discussing the possibility of carrying out a mental capacity assessment, HSWs tended to intimate that a better knowledge of, and a closer relationship with, the patient than they had would be needed. The idea that a professional needs to know a person well to be able to do a capacity assessment is not contained within the Mental Capacity Act 2005. While there might be an advantage to knowing someone reasonably well before undertaking an assessment in order to be familiar with how they communicate, it would be perfectly possible even for a stranger to follow the prescribed formula and establish with reasonable confidence a person's mental capacity with regards to a given decision (Department for Constitutional Affairs, 2007). The HSWs' insistence on deferring to doctors for mental capacity assessments in most instances might be understood as a strategy that was useful for managing their already high work load and for avoiding situations of uncertainty and dilemma. Lipsky (1980) argues that this is a common practice employed by street level bureaucrats to make their work more predictable and manageable. In light of the high demand for HSW services and the pressure from managers and clinician colleagues to expedite discharges as quickly as possible, such practices are understandable.

Discretion can be used by HSWs either to manipulate the bureaucratic system in favour of a patient, or to develop practices that make their work-load more manageable and predictable. The bureaucratic system in which they work relies on HSWs to carry out their work independently until the point where a care plan is presented for approval, meaning that some discretion will always be present. Where the discretion of HSWs touches on the managerial priority of swift patient discharges, it is relatively limited and can be easily checked by managerial intervention. By contrast, practices which relate more to the quality of a HSW's intervention, such as lack of involvement in the complex and uncertain assessment of mental capacity, are allowed to develop freely, so that they appear to take on the concrete form of a deliberate policy.

Conclusion

This chapter has explored the nature of the bureaucratic systems in which the HSWs practise. HSWs are subject to extensive managerial control which encourages Fordist and Taylorist approaches to practice and the dehumanisation of patients as a means of enabling their swift and efficient discharge from hospital. This does not imply that HSWs should be regarded only as bureaucrats, or that they adopt the officiousness and inhumanity commonly associated with bureaucracy (Payne, 2000). Indeed, the humanitarian professional values of the HSWs and their efforts to enable patients to become empowered will be explored in the next chapter. Despite managerial control, there remains space in their work for HSWs to employ discretion. While sometimes this discretion is exercised with the purpose of making their work more manageable, there are also instances of HSWs explicitly using discretion in the interests of the patient in direct opposition to the managerial emphasis on the speedy discharge of patients. The bureaucratic and managerial systems are therefore only partially successful in controlling social work practice, both because they still allow some room for discretion, and because they are not fully able to oblige or convince HSWs to prioritise efficiency over all other considerations in their work.

6 Is it still social work?

Introduction

The previous chapter highlighted the constraints and pressures that control and limit social work practice within the hospital. The bureaucratic nature of the routine tasks the HSWs perform, the pressure from hospital management and local authority senior managers to expedite patient discharges with speed, and the demands of maintaining a working space alongside the hierarchy of hospital professionals mean that the hospital is a uniquely challenging environment for social work practice. Despite these challenges, the HSWs involved in this study still consider the work they do to be 'social work'. Using the International Federation of Social Workers' (IFSW, 2014) global definition of social work as a starting point for analysis, this chapter will examine the extent to which HSWs' work can be recognised as social work, exploring the values that HSWs articulate and enact in their work. Particular attention will be paid to the HSWs' claim to be advocates for patients and carers (see also Chapter 7) and the nature of the relationship between HSWs and those who rely on their services. It will be argued that HSWs are able to do work that is recognisable as social work, including some examples of challenging structural disadvantage at a personal level, but that it is not possible for them to fulfil the ambitious aims espoused by more radical interpretations of the social work role (e.g. Dominelli, 2002; Rogowski, 2010; Ife, 2012). It will be suggested, however, that the deficit lies in the ideas, which do not match the realities of statutory social work more widely, rather than in the practices of HSWs specifically. Despite the HSWs' orientation towards the empowerment of patients and carers, this chapter will note that their practices perpetuate their own professional power by preserving their exclusive right to define social care needs and plan care.

The IFSW (2014) defines social work thus:

> Social work is a practice-based profession and an academic discipline that promotes social change and development, social cohesion, and the empowerment and liberation of people. Principles of social justice, human rights, collective responsibility and respect for diversities are

central to social work. Underpinned by theories of social work, social sciences, humanities and indigenous knowledges, social work engages people and structures to address life challenges and enhance wellbeing.

The work of HSWs does not often give rise to opportunities to engage at the macro or even meso levels of interactions between individuals and society. However, in claiming the role of advocacy (see Chapter 7, and below), HSWs within this study demonstrated an ambition to be involved with the empowerment and liberation of the individual people who use their services. Further, the allocation of resources through care planning touches on social justice, human rights and collective responsibility, while respect for diversity is a core concern for social workers in a multi-cultural country such as the UK (Thompson, 2016). The IFSW definition is therefore relevant to the work of HSWs, and assessment of their practices against the definition can reveal the extent to which they engage in social work, as opposed to ful-filling their bureaucratic functions without concern for the principles and practices that lie at the heart of social work. This chapter will consider in depth two aspects of the IFSW definition that appear to have direct rele-vance to HSW practice: human rights and social justice, before moving on to explore empowerment in the context of the advocacy role HSWs claim for themselves (see Chapter 7).

This chapter's emphasis on examination of the HSWs' practices regarding human rights, social justice and empowerment rests on the premise that these principles are a sine qua non of social work. All three values are noted to be central to the formulation of critical gerontological social work prac-tice (Ray et al., 2009), which takes social work with older people beyond the operation of bureaucracy to address issues of discrimination and oppression in their lives. As noted in Chapter 2, UK social work can trace its historical roots to two main strands: the Charity Organisation Society, which gave rise to the more conservative strand of 'casework', based on helping the indivi-dual to learn to cope better with the world, and the Settlements movement, which took a more structural approach to understanding and alleviating human distress. Statutory social work tends to owe more to the 'casework' approach, in which assistance is offered at the individual level, yet under-standing of the structural causes of social problems remains an integral part of social work education and, even in statutory roles, social workers main-tain a commitment to the principles of human rights, social justice and empowerment (Hugman, 2009). All of these principles revolve around addressing issues of power differentials, which are of central importance to anti-oppressive practice (Dominelli, 2002). Anti-oppressiveness has become a unifying ideology within social work (Millar, 2008), and lies at the centre of emancipatory approaches that are seen understood as the core of modern social work (Thompson, 2015). Proponents of anti-oppressive practice argue that social workers have an obligation to address not only the power differ-entials they encounter at the individual level, but also those that arise within larger social structures and processes (Dominelli, 2002). This chapter therefore will be concerned not only with the extent to which HSWs are able to promote human rights, social justice and empowerment at the level of the individual, but also with the extent to which HSWs engage with the larger social structures at play for the patients and carers with whom they are concerned.

Power differentials often arise due to individuals' belonging to social groups that are disadvantaged, such as women, people of minority ethnic backgrounds, people who are disabled, people who are poor, and people who are non-heterosexual or non-cisgender (Thompson, 2016). Not all of these social categories are mentioned in the chapter below, since the HSWs' patients within this study tended to be older people who are predominantly white, working or middle class and heterosexual. An attempt to frame the discussion of HSWs' responses around all the various forms of discrimination would therefore impose an artificial structure on the data that were gathered.

The discussions that follow should be read with the understanding that HSWs demonstrate a deep personal commitment to their patients always in mind. Striking about the way HSWs approached their work during the fieldwork was their empathy for both patients and carers. This was frequently expressed when their views were elicited both in formal interviews and conversations. For example, two social workers were discussing the pressure that patients sometimes experience from family members to go into residential care and one commented,

> If people were trying to make decisions for me and I had capacity I'd be sitting there wanting to scream.
>
> (Fieldnote – HSW2)

Empathy for patients is not confined to HSWs' discussions of their work, however, but also colours their interactions with colleagues within the hospital. During a telephone call with a nurse regarding a patient whose false teeth had been lost, for example, another HSW commented,

> I mean, if that were my mother I'd put in a pretty strong complaint.
>
> (Fieldnote – HSW3)

The willingness of HSWs to imagine themselves in the position of patients or carers is a powerful counterweight to the dehumanising procedures and practices discussed in Chapter 5. Empathy is significant in social work because it moves beyond an emotive or cognitive response to a person or situation to provoking a conscious decision to take informed action (Gerdes and Segal, 2009). Thus, by cultivating a sense of empathy in their work, HSWs make a conscious personal commitment to the well-being of patients and carers, which may encourage an orientation towards the social work values of human rights, social justice and empowerment (Payne, 2014).

Human rights

It is interesting that no explicit mention of or reference to the Human Rights Act 1998 was recorded during either the fieldwork or interviews, despite HSWs' concern for individual self-determination. This suggests that the legal framework underpinning the human rights of patients, which HSWs are concerned to uphold, holds far less sway than their conception of individual rights as arising as an implicit component of human nature (Ife, 2010). The right of the individual to self-determination appears to be the most prominent human right with which the HSWs are concerned. During fieldwork and interviews, this was frequently expressed in terms of the choices and decisions patients might make, for example:

> [A]nyway, it's his choice to live like that, and he's got the right to make that choice. Even if it's a bad choice, he's got capacity so it's his choice.
>
> (Fieldnote – HSW4)

> Well, if somebody's got capacity, they make their own decisions.
>
> (Interview – HSW5)

It is striking that HSWs' discussions regarding the rights of patients to self-determination are often subject to the proviso that the patient has the necessary mental capacity to make decisions. The frequency with which mental capacity is mentioned when related to patients' choices is understandable in light of the frequency with which HSWs are involved with people of limited mental capacity due to both long-term conditions such as dementia and the short-term effects of physical illness. In terms of the European Convention on Human Rights, the type of self-determination with which HSWs show concern incorporates Article 5 – the right to liberty – and Article 8 – the right to privacy, family life, home and correspondence. While the HSWs' frequent use of the term 'choice' recalls the language of neoliberalism, with its emphasis on consumer choice (Beckett and Maynard, 2013), 'choice' should here be understood in terms of the decisions self-determining individuals make about their lives, rather than the selections of welfare goods by a customer.

Self-determination as understood by the HSWs can be defined as a negative right, as it is the right to be free from interference, as opposed to a positive right, in which an active effort might be made to enable people to enhance their self-determination (Banks, 2012). The emphasis on negative rights in HSWs' priorities can be seen in HSWs' willingness to support patients whose mental capacity is not in doubt to make decisions that they might consider unwise. Such a stance can be uncomfortable for the HSWs when they perceive that a '*bad choice*' will lead to the patient suffering:

> I had this man who just refused to have a care package. He hated social workers – he'd had his kids removed, his daughter had had her kids

removed and all that. I'd talk to him and he just wouldn't take any notice of a word I'd say... He wasn't safe to go home but just refused a package of care, so I made him sign a disclaimer in the end to say he was going home without a package of care against my recommendation... I don't know where he is now. I've rung his GP to tell him I'm concerned but there's not a lot more I can do. I do wonder where he is now.

(Fieldnote – HSW4)

Before accepting the man's refusal of a package of care, the HSW did his best to follow a model of positive rights promotion, spending a considerable amount of time on attempting to build a rapport with the man so that he would accept support through social services. Though he was unsuccessful in persuading the man to accept a package of care, the HSW did gain his trust enough that he allowed him to liaise with other agencies and professionals on his behalf, meaning that he was able to assist with an issue related to his housing tenancy. The HSW also sought other avenues of support for him through family members and through a tenancy support worker. The HSW's contact with the GP indicates his reluctance to leave the man in an unsafe and distressing situation. Ultimately, however, though the HSW attempted to promote social justice through raising the man's awareness of his rights, adherence to the principle of self-determination as a right to be free from interference took priority.

While self-determination might be taken as the most important human right to the HSWs, it is not the only human right with which HSWs show concern. Even if they do not express their concerns within the discourse of human rights, HSWs involved in identifying and responding to the abuse or neglect of vulnerable adults are concerned with human rights including property rights, freedom from torture and servitude, and freedom of conscience and religion (Mantell, 2011). In such cases, the HSWs work alongside a POVA (protection of vulnerable adults) team within the local authority, who co-ordinate investigations. During the fieldwork, for example, one HSW had identified suspected abuse and referred to the POVA team, and once this referral was made, her main involvement in the investigation process was to search through medical files for some photographs of injuries that were meant to have been taken as evidence for the investigation. HSWs continue to do face-to-face work with patients whose circumstances are subject to a safeguarding investigation, and may interview such patients regarding the concerns if appropriate, but decisions about safeguarding issues are taken by the POVA team. Regarding a patient about whom there was a safeguarding concern, one HSW was heard to comment during a telephone call,

Well POVA have to do their investigation ... She's safe for now and all her needs are met, but yeah, I think she's going to have to go into placement ...

(Fieldnote – HSW4)

The HSW's analysis of the overall situation for the patient could only be provisional until the outcome of the POVA investigation. Thus, the HSWs' promotion of human rights takes place within a wider bureaucracy in which defined procedures have to be enacted in response to identified needs. This fragmentation of the social work role could be perceived as disempowering to the HSWs, since they are forced to rely on the actions and decisions of another team, yet HSWs value the system because it affords an extra layer of protection to people's human rights by ensuring that abuse is properly investigated by a team that is not subject to the same pressures regarding the swift discharge of patients.

While the HSWs can be said to show a concern for protecting human rights, their involvement with people whose mental capacity is in doubt means that they often have to deal with situations in which people's right to self-determination is denied to them. In such situations, the Mental Capacity Act 2005 requires all professionals and carers involved to act in the best interests of the person lacking capacity. HSWs have a crucial part to play in seeking and documenting the consensus of professionals and carers over the care plans that must be made.

> If they haven't got capacity then we would make sure there's a formal capacity assessment completed and we would have a Best Interest Meeting then with professionals and family to see what is the best discharge destination for that individual.
>
> (Interview – HSW1)

As discussed in Chapters 5 and 7, HSWs often leave formal assessment of capacity to doctors, but are willing to take the responsibility if they do not agree with doctors' assessments. HSWs can be vehement in their insistence that the capacity assessments of doctors be properly documented and that patients should always be included in meetings unless capacity prevents them:

> I've got a man up on Ward __ who's been treated appallingly. They say they've done a capacity assessment but there isn't one in the file. And then apparently he's got behavioural issues but there's no behaviour charts in the files.
>
> (Fieldnote – HSW4)

While HSWs do not regularly draw on the legislative framework of human rights in their approach to patients who have capacity, their consideration for the human rights of people deemed to lack capacity is heavily bound up with their understanding of the requirements of the Mental Capacity Act 2005. Thus, while the negative freedoms of human rights are considered by HSWs to be natural rights, their removal can only be sanctioned by HSWs within the context of specific legislation. The emotive language used by the HSW reflects his personal commitment to the rights of the patient. His portrayal of the practices on the ward in question as appalling to the patient personally, rather than as simply an example of poor practice in general, reflects an empathic awareness that the actions of clinicians would have a material impact on the human rights of the patient. It should be noted, however, that the HSWs keep their responses to perceived injustices such as the above example at the personal level. Though he was concerned at the treatment the patient had been receiving, as long as he was able to ensure that this patient's rights would now be respected, there was no suggestion that he would take his complaint further, even to the level of management. He thus avoided politicising this as a human rights issue by not considering action to challenge the perceived injustice at a higher level (Ife, 2012).

As well as promoting the legal rights of patients deemed to lack capacity, HSWs consider human rights through their concern for establishing what is really in the best interests of the patient. Regarding the decision-making process for one patient deemed to lack capacity who might need residential care, one HSW commented:

> It's a difficult one. We know she'll be safer in a residential home, but it might make her miserable...
>
> (Fieldnote – HSW5)

In considering the patient's potential happiness in the home that might be provided for her, the HSW is considering her right to a home and her right to security, while the consideration of her safety touches on her right to life – i.e. Articles 8, 5 and 2 respectively of the European Convention on Human Rights. It is perhaps encouraging to note that the HSW's concern for the patient's happiness might suggest that the assessed inability of the patient to make her own decision removes an element of her human rights, but does not diminish her humanity in the eyes of the HSW.

In so far as they are concerned with promoting the self-determination of individual patients, and with ensuring their right to life, security and freedom from torture or degrading treatment, HSWs can claim to be promoting human rights. The promotion of human rights by the HSWs is often couched in the language of individual choice, yet this reflects a preoccupation with a broad sense of self-determination, rather than a simple consumer choice between services in a marketplace. Generally, human rights are viewed by the HSWs as natural rights, and only when they are to be removed do HSWs rely on legislation to guide their practice. The principle of individuals' self-determination appears to be fundamental to the HSWs' practice, and is understood as a deontological imperative. The HSWs' regard for human rights tends to be limited to the individual level, and does not lead them to take overtly political action to address wider issues of structure.

Social justice

Social justice, understood as the fair distribution of benefits and rewards throughout society (Heywood, 2004) is at the core of the aspirations of social work (Clark, 2000). As with human rights, the bureaucratic nature of their daily tasks means that HSWs are not in a position to campaign for social justice at the meso or macro level, in terms of seeking structural or political changes that might result in fairer distribution of wealth, opportunities and privilege for the disadvantaged or oppressed, as advocated by modern proponents of a radical form of social work (e.g. Dominelli, 2002; Rogowski, 2010; Ife, 2012). Work towards social justice can, however, be seen in the way HSWs seek to improve the lives of patients through their care planning. In an interview, one HSW described effusively the satisfaction she felt in seeing the well-being of a patient improve after complex negotiations with her relatives eventually resulted in her finding permanent accommodation in a residential home:

> I mean, she's being cared for, she's made a really good recovery, she's eating and drinking in her nursing home, the manager says she's much happier... She's happier now she sees all of the children and now she's seeing her family, great-grandchildren she's never seen before... This woman has absolutely blossomed since she's gone in... And to see her actually improving to what she was on the ward is well worth the effort. Because I know she's safe and being looked after.
>
> (Interview – HSW1)

For older people facing declining physical and mental health, access to appropriate care and opportunities to maintain family relationships are vital issues (Age UK, 2011). Arranging the most appropriate care plan for a patient therefore promotes social justice by giving a person access to the resources most likely to promote her/his happiness. The sincere concern of the HSW for the happiness of the patient is indicative of a person-centred approach (Kitwood, 1997) that is concerned with more than the efficiency of the bureaucratic function of moving patients out of hospital beds. By arranging a care plan that is successful in enabling the happiness of an individual, a HSW does not overtly challenge injustice or change society for the better, but she does have a part in enabling an individual to benefit from collective responsibility for the welfare of individuals.

Commitment to issues of social justice can also be seen in HSWs' concern to ensure fairness in the access of patients to the HSW service. While many HSWs acknowledged the difficulties arising from not having allocated wards on which to work – which means HSWs are unable to sustain long-term working relationships with clinicians – they also asserted that the system is fairer to patients because waiting times do not vary for patients depending on which ward they are staying in. Similarly, there is concern for fair allocation of resources. Concerning a patient who was repeatedly admitted to the hospital for fabricated symptoms, who appeared to want to go into residential care but had hitherto refused to submit to a financial assessment to determine whether or not she should self-fund, HSW3 commented to a fellow team member that it might save time and money if the local authority and NHS trust simply agreed to fund residential care for her. Her immediate response was to point out,

But what about all the other patients in need? How is that fair to them?
(Fieldnote – HSW5)

As was noted in Chapter 5, there is an ethical obligation on HSWs to ensure that publicly funded resources are distributed as fairly as possible. Social justice for the HSWs implies not only that people should have opportunities for happiness, but also that those who have the means to support themselves should pay. Thus, there is an underlying communitarian belief in the balance of rights and obligations (Giddens, 1998). (It will be noted in Chapter 7 that the HSWs sometimes show resistance to clinicians' ways of gatekeeping NHS resources with regard to Continuing Healthcare funding. This dissonance can perhaps be explained by the HSWs not understanding the criteria upon which clinicians base their decisions.) The comment made by HSW5 here would suggest that, as with the right of individuals to self-determination noted above, the balance between rights and responsibilities is interpreted in a deontological rather than utilitarian way by the HSWs. An unequal distribution of resources in favour of this particular patient might ultimately result in time and money being saved by both the hospital and the local authority, as well as greatly enhancing her well-being, yet the HSWs ruled this out because unequal treatment was viewed as wrong.

While the above patient's case illustrates the commitment of the HSWs to some aspects of social justice, it also illustrates the limitations which restrict their ability to work towards it. Frequent fabrication of symptoms of physical illness is suggestive of unmet psychological, emotional or social need (Bass and Halligan, 2014). The patient was assessed by a psychiatrist and deemed ineligible for mental health services, but was clearly in need of more support than could be supplied through the standard HSW process of an assessment and care plan to meet basic physical care needs. The HSW's inability to provide a service to the patient beyond the usual bureaucratic functions thus was likely to result in a continued lack of opportunity for her to live a fulfilling life. The services this patient needed to overcome her difficulties were not available, yet the HSW did not challenge the lack of services, whether through raising consciousness or linking her with others in a similar situation. The emphasis on bureaucratic functions noted in Chapter 5 therefore has a limiting impact on HSWs' ability to promote social justice.

Despite the emphasis on bureaucratic functions, there are times when HSWs act within the hospital to safeguard social justice at the personal level. It was noted in Chapter 5 that HSWs sometimes improvise outside their bureaucratic role to support the smooth operation of services for a patient. One such improvisation noted during fieldwork was clearly rooted in the personal concern of the HSW for an individual patient who was at risk of disadvantage through poor services:

HSW4: I've just had a phone call from patient flow. They've moved one of
    mine from __ Ward to __ Ward but his Zimmer frame's been left behind.
HSW1: He'll be in pads[1] by the end of the week.

HSW2: Or he'll be on the steady,[2] look.
HSW4: No, I told them I'm coming up and I'm going to sort that out.
(Fieldnote)

The personal responsibility that HSW4 assumed for finding the patient's Zimmer frame was emphasised in his repeated use of 'I' in the last sentence. His actions serve social justice by making sure that the patient retains access to the equipment that may prevent him from becoming more disabled. Though the HSW's actions appear fairly insignificant, they reflect a concern that was expressed by many HSWs during the fieldwork: that patients' physical abilities decline during hospital admissions due to the lack of appropriate care on the wards. Hospital admissions often have a drastic impact on older people's mobility (National Audit Office, 2016) and many of the HSWs felt that this was exacerbated by practices on the wards which save time for nurses and health care assistants, such as using a steady to transfer a patient to the toilet instead of taking the extra time to support them to walk there. The HSWs' concerns regarding the care of older people in hospitals is corroborated by recent research. Calnan et al. (2013) found hospital systems do not prioritise patients' dignity and that the physical environments of acute hospital wards are unsuited to older people. Further, Hillman et al. (2013) found that the risk reduction priorities of hospital systems result in disadvantages for patients through dehumanising standard procedures (e.g. around patient isolation to prevent the spread of infection) and the risk-averse practices of individual clinicians. Regarding one ward where poor care was felt to be particularly endemic, a HSW in this study commented,

> The lack of rehabilitation, it's sad really. Some of the practices I've seen have made me wonder if I should be referring them to POVA.
> (Fieldnote – HSW1)

The perceived paucity of rehabilitation services is an issue of social justice, particularly since many older people struggle to speak up for themselves because of frailty, disability and stigma (Ray et al., 2009). It is striking that, though some of the HSWs felt this concern, they did not take the action of following POVA procedures or seeking change through expressing concerns to higher managers. As was noted with possible human rights violations above, the HSWs are unwilling to move beyond remedying the situation at the personal level. While, during conversations over lunch and breaks, the HSWs would discuss the political context of 'austerity' cuts to public services, and their own local authority's policy on developing the town centre while cutting spending on social care, they did not tend to apply their political views to the individual patients they encountered. It would appear that the sensitivities of social workers to issues of human rights and social justice are keen, yet their power to agitate for these at a level beyond the personal is minimal

(Ferguson, 2007). This would suggest that the bureaucratic separation of practice from the moral implications of practice (see Chapter 5) has the effect of separating the personal from the political in the world view of the HSWs.

While the HSWs show concern for social justice in their practice at the personal level, it is apparent that social justice takes a lower priority for them than self-determination. This can be seen in the non-judgemental stance HSWs take towards the ways in which patients exercise their freedom. An example of this arose in discussion of an inpatient who was discovered to be giving away money to his friends and spending substantial amounts on the services of prostitutes. The nursing staff sought to question his mental capacity, yet as this was not in doubt, the HSW involved was clear that no action could, or should, be taken to prevent his continuing to spend his money in this way. Her pragmatic comment:

> At least he's spent it on something he enjoys…
>
> (Fieldnote – HSW7)

demonstrates the extent to which the HSWs avoid moral judgement and place emphasis on the freedom of individuals to decide on their own actions. From a position of respect for the self-determination of the individual, there is no difficulty with the HSW's stance here. The non-judgemental stance, however, does result in the HSW taking a neutral stance towards prostitution – a practice which research evidence suggests brings to women 'even greater poverty, social ostracism, exploitation, abuse, housing difficulties, dependence on men…' (Phoenix, 1999, p. 100). Of course, there are alternative perspectives that emphasise the agency of women involved in prostitution and advocate for the freedom of women to use their own bodies as they see fit (Leigh, 2004). For an occupation that claims to support liberation and social justice (IFSW, 2014), however, a neutral position towards the patient's use of prostitutes – in which the perspective of the prostitute is not considered – appears to be contradictory.

In their role as gatekeepers of social care services, HSWS, as with all social workers involved in planning community care, have a part to play in promoting social justice. HSWs show a concern for fairness in terms of how their services are distributed, and operate the mechanisms of bureaucracy in ways that enable individuals to have access to opportunities for personal fulfilment. They also show willingness to improvise outside their bureaucratic role in order to protect individuals from becoming disabled by services that are inappropriate or even neglectful. The HSWs do not operate beyond the personal level, however, e.g. by challenging disadvantages they discover either through approved mechanisms such as POVA or through involvement in wider agitations or consciousness-raising. While they are able to be critical in their understanding of the disadvantages the users of their services may encounter, the nature of their role as statutory social workers limits their practice to the micro level.

Advocacy and empowerment

Empowerment should be understood not as something that can be given by a professional to an individual or group, but as a condition that a person is able to achieve through her/his own actions (Lymbery, 2005). Where social workers seek to promote empowerment, they should therefore be understood to be working to create or support the conditions under which empowerment is possible (Ray and Phillips, 2012). It is possible for HSWs facilitate empowerment when they produce care plans that are tailored towards the choices that patients wish to make about their lives. For such empowerment to occur, HSWs embrace the role of advocates for patients. As will be discussed further in Chapter 7, the role of patient advocate is central to HSWs' self-perception and their understanding of how they relate to clinicians within the hospital. While, as has been noted above, HSWs do not readily engage in agitations to create a fairer society or to correct structural injustices, the self-assumed position of advocate allows HSWs to feel that they are challenging the powerful on behalf of the powerless:

> If it wasn't for us advocating, people would be caught up in the process and their choices would be forgotten about.
>
> (Fieldnote – HSW2)

It is interesting that the HSW regards discharge planning as a process in which the wishes of a patient can easily be forgotten about. This suggests an understanding of the bureaucratic systems of both the hospital and the local authority as disempowering to patients. In casting themselves as advocates for patients, HSWs' aim is not only for the patient's voice to be heard, but for their wishes to be enacted by the services involved. This distinguishes HSWs from the independent advocates provided by some voluntary sector agencies (e.g. Age Cymru), whose purpose is only to ensure that the views of an individual are heard and noted within decision-making processes. By contrast, the advocacy of the HSWs would appear to fit the definition supplied by Sosin and Caulum (1983, p. 13):

> An attempt, having a greater than zero probability of success, by an individual or group to influence another individual or group to make a decision that would not have been made otherwise and that concerns the welfare or interests of a third party who is in a less powerful status than the decision maker.

It might appear contradictory that HSWs could fit this definition of advocates when they themselves are often decision-makers, since they are responsible for submitting care plans in order to secure resources for patients. This contradiction is solved by a full consideration of the primacy of patients' or (when patients are deemed to lack capacity) carers' wishes in the HSWs' assessment processes. In carrying out an assessment, typically HSWs do not regard themselves as having expert knowledge as to the patient's needs, and therefore they do not consider their own opinion to be final. As noted in Chapter 7, expert knowledge regarding patients' medical needs is supplied through clinicians, yet this knowledge is used only to ascertain a patient's eligibility for services, not what services the patient ends up receiving. The wishes of the patient or carer(s) are at the centre of the HSWs' assessment and care plan. The care plan that the HSW produces is the result of an attempt to match what the patient/carer(s) wants with what their medical need makes eligible and what any involved informal carers might be willing to support. Advocacy on behalf of patients, therefore, is most often concerned with persuading a patient's family members, or persuading professionals, to respect the wishes of the patient. Since the patient's desired outcome is therefore achieved through the deeds of the HSW rather than the agency of the patient, it is possible to argue that empowerment does not occur. Ultimately, however, if a decision has been taken by a patient and then enacted by the HSW, the HSW can be regarded as the instrument of the patient's will.

The need for HSWs to act as advocates with family members can arise because of the discovery of abuse or neglect, but often arises because family members have innocent but set ideas about the kind of care they want for the patient. The power of family members was frequently referred to by the HSWs.

HSW1: I have a patient who has capacity, movement and continence but risk of falls and she's being assessed for residential. She's told me she wants to go home, but says to me, 'Don't tell my daughter'. But I said to her, 'Should we be planning for you to go home? If that's what you want, I can talk to your daughter about it.' And eventually she agreed to talk to her daughter, but it was hard for her because her daughter wanted her in residential.

HSW2: Families can be so powerful all coming together.

(Fieldnote)

Wanting the best for a patient very often means that family members want to see them physically safe, and err on the side of caution in suggesting care plans that would reduce the patient's independence. As HSW2 notes, families can hold high levels of power over elderly people who are ill and frail, such that, as in this case, the individual feels unable to speak up for her own independence. In a society in which older people are marginalised rather than valued, ideas of old age as encompassing helplessness and passivity permeate each generation (Pickard, 2016; Ray and Phillips, 2012). In encouraging the patient to speak up for what she wants to happen, the HSW therefore challenges an oppressive culture and assists the patient's liberation and empowerment. It has been suggested (e.g. Rose, 1990; Pullen-Sansfacon and Cowden, 2012) that empowerment involves not only putting the viewpoint of a less powerful individual or group forward, but also raising their consciousness of the social context in which they are rendered powerless and the true range of choices that may be open to them. In the example above, the HSW can certainly be said to have raised the patient's understanding of the choices open to her. It may also be the case that through her interaction with the HSW, the patient's awareness of her family's ageist assumptions was raised.

The advocacy provided by the HSWs often revolves around the discourse of risk. During the fieldwork, the HSWs' orientation towards risk varied depending on the situation. Often, as described above, the HSWs would advocate for positive risk-taking – weighing the benefits of taking a risk against the negatives of not taking it (Morgan, 1996). When advocating positive risks, the HSWs tend to regard even small successes as worthy of effort. For example, describing a care plan for which she had advocated, which had lasted for six months before the individual concerned had to be admitted again to hospital following a fall, one HSW commented,

> So to me that was an achievement, that was really good, so she'd done really well.
>
> (Interview – HSW9)

The individual involved had been diagnosed with dementia and was physically frail, so it was likely that she would reach the point where going into residential care would be inevitable. In her willingness to facilitate the patient's wish to remain at home for as long as possible, however, the HSW placed respect for the patient's right to self-determination above the most efficient and lowest-risk option, which would have been to press her to accept earlier placement in residential care.

By contrast, the discourse of risk can also be used by HSWs as a means of advocating against professionals putting patients' safety in jeopardy by discharging too hastily. In an interview, a ward sister commented on HSWs' unwillingness to take risks with patients' safety:

> I do think a lot of our decisions are made without the risks being weighed up, to be honest… We go, nurses, sometimes very close to the wind. But if a social worker is involved, they don't take risks… I'll say yes, the social worker will say no.
>
> (Interview – Ward Sister 2)

HSWs support risks that patients wish to take in making decisions about their own lives, but act against clinicians who wish to risk a patient's safety in order to free a bed for the next patient. This demonstrates that the loyalties of HSWs lie firmly with the individual patient. The ability of HSWs to 'say no', acknowledged by the ward sister, suggests that HSWs wield real power on behalf of patients. Wielding such power could not be said to be empowering to patients, since they are not included in the decision-making, but it does serve to protect patients from disadvantage and further curtailment of their liberty through incurring further injury or illness as a result of premature discharge.

That HSWs are able to provoke a sense of empowerment through advocacy can be seen in the words of patients and carers. When asked who makes decisions about his care, one patient interviewed during fieldwork expressed a firm belief in his own self-determination.

> She answered my questions and was very clear – if you don't want to do it, don't do it... the decisions are made by the three of us: me, my son and my daughter-in-law. But nothing would be done against my will.
>
> (Interview – Patient 1)

This patient had recently agreed to be discharged from hospital into a residential placement for short-term physical rehabilitation, which would then lead to him returning to his own home. The patient's confidence that nothing would be done against his will reflects his trust in his relatives and the professionals involved, but also demonstrates a strong sense of empowerment. His repetition of the HSW's words suggests that her interaction with him had an effect in creating this sense of empowerment. The knowledge about both the available services and his rights that the patient appears to have gained from his HSW enable him to participate fully in the planning of his care (Adams, 2008). This demonstrates that advocacy is not a fiction created by HSWs in order to feel that they are still doing 'social work' even in a highly bureaucratised role, but a practice that can have a tangible impact on the lives of patients and carers.

The impact of HSWs as advocates was even more evident in the words of carers interviewed during the fieldwork. Carers reported emotional benefits of having a HSW to advocate on their behalf within the hospital:

> So HSW2, basically she became our advocate for the family because there was still pressure from people within the hospital to say why aren't you just taking him home? And HSW2 was able to say, no I had a conversation and he was very clear about what he wanted, and this is the way we're going to be working.
>
> (Interview – Carer 1)

> [W]here you feel like you're up against a battle, I have somebody to shield me from it a bit because at least she can fight our corner.
>
> (Interview – Carer 2)

The sense of relief carers expressed at having a HSW often related to having someone to assist them in expressing opposing views to clinicians and dealing with conflict about what should happen to a patient – especially in situations in which it was agreed that the patient did not have capacity to make their own decisions. The practice of the HSWs can therefore be seen in the light of addressing the power differentials between health care professionals and carers (Johnson, 1972; Larson, 1977). The advocacy HSWs offer sometimes involves empowering people to speak for themselves, but also sometimes involves speaking on their behalf to ensure that their decisions are enacted.

While it is clear that the HSWs are able to support empowerment through advocacy, there is one aspect of advocacy in which their practice might be thought to be weak. Advocacy involves not only ensuring that an individual or group is heard and is respected within a decision-making process, but also in ensuring that the individual or group is supported to grasp the range of choices available to them (Rose, 1990). While HSWs are able to make patients and carers aware of the types of provision that are available and the outline of what a care plan might be, they are not able to facilitate a consumer-type choice between the services available. For care in the home, a 'brokerage' team arranges the care agreed in the HSW's plan without any input from the patient (or the HSW) in selection of the provider (see Chapter 4). In the case of choosing a residential home, the HSWs are unable to give information or opinions to patients or carers about the standard of care provided in any of the available options, on the grounds that this might leave them open to accusations of bribery or detriment to the business of ill-favoured providers. This leads to a situation in which HSWs are all but powerless to promote the best interests of the individual going into residential care. One HSW commented about a former patient who seemed depressed since moving into residential care:

> Well I'd be depressed if I had to live in that room. And he's only a young guy – maybe in his 70s, so he could be facing 20 years in that room!... I wrote in his file that he needs to go to a better room as soon as one becomes available. And I told his son to keep on top of that.
>
> (Fieldnote – HSW5)

This is a typical example of a type of conversation that took place regularly among the HSWs during the fieldwork – the HSWs had strong opinions about some care homes, but were not able to influence carers or patients overtly in their choices. The empathy and personal concern of the HSW for the well-being of the patient is once again evident, yet the HSW does not consider any action beyond the personal level – in this case, encouraging the patient's son to be proactive after her involvement has ended. This means that the market system on which community care now relies is far less effective than it could be in maintaining standards, since competition between the goods available is not facilitated by a fair and open market. While local authorities keep lists of approved care homes, which are updated when information is provided by social care professionals (e.g. community care management social workers, Deprivation of Liberty assessors, POVA investigators etc.), and while there is a regime of care home inspection, the recent discovery of widespread neglect and abuse in care homes (Greener, 2015) would suggest that these mechanisms are not enough. It is therefore once again evident that the HSWs do not feel able to engage in activities to raise awareness of structural disadvantage or to agitate for change in society, even at a local level.

Inasmuch as the practices of HSWs are orientated towards human rights, social justice and empowerment, albeit predominantly at the individual level, their values might be understood as 'modern, emancipatory values' (Lishman et al., 2018, p. 9). An assumption of such values is that the social worker should not be regarded as an expert with an implicit right to diagnose the cause of an individual's difficulties and the necessary treatment, as is the case in the traditional 'medical model' (Laing, 1971), but that social worker and the user of services should be regarded as partners working together. Despite their emancipatory leanings, however, the HSWs retain some elements of professional power. Their role as gatekeepers of services arises from their power to define need in the assessment and care planning process, and with the ability to define needs comes some control of discourse and therefore power (Foucault, [1975] 1991). The intentional retention of power by HSWs can be seen in one HSW's comment to an independent advocate about their role:

> HSW3 asks the representative of the advocacy service what she would do if a patient deemed to have capacity expressed a wish to do something dangerous. The representative replies that she would still have to advocate for them, as long as they have capacity. HSW4 comments that he would not 'take kindly' to this sort of intervention if he could see that a discharge home would fail, adding that risk assessment is part of the social work role.
>
> (Fieldnote)

HSW4's emphasis on the risk assessment role serves to underline his own expertise, and therefore the inappropriateness of challenging his recommendations. It is ironic that HSWs place so much emphasis on their own advocacy role, yet feel so wary of advocates from outside their service. This reflects how HSWs must balance more than one moral imperative at a time: the emphasis on empowerment and choice must be balanced with appropriate management of risks.

The fieldwork suggested that the advocacy role is at the heart of HSWs' practices, and that their advocacy can make a tangible difference to the lives of patients and carers. HSWs act as advocates both on behalf of patients towards family members and on behalf of patients and carers to clinicians. There is some evidence of a critical approach towards environments and practices that disempower older people (Ray et al., 2009) and attempts to make empowerment possible, even if HSWs must sometimes act as the instruments of patients' or carers' will, rather than enabling a direct exchange of power. A theme running through discussion of HSWs' contribution to human rights and social justice also found in the discussion of advocacy and empowerment, however, is that the HSWs do not work beyond the level of the individual to advocate for wider changes in society. Unsurprisingly in a statutory role, the practices of the HSWs might therefore be understood as comprising a conservative form of social work, aimed at mitigating the disadvantages arising from neoliberalism (Ferguson, 2007; Rogowski, 2010), without challenging the social and structural disadvantages underlying individual difficulties.

Conclusion

This chapter has explored the extent to which the work of HSWs can still be said to be 'social work' as understood in the IFSW (2014) global definition. It has been possible to detect in the HSWs' practices orientation towards values commonly regarded as central to social work practice: human rights, social justice and empowerment. The ambitions of HSWs in response to these values are conservative, however, reflecting their descent from the 'casework' tradition. HSWs work at the personal level to promote social justice and patients' and carers' human rights and their advocacy has tangible benefits to patients and carers, yet they do not tend to undertake practices aimed at changing the wider social and structural causes of the disadvantages they encounter. To do so would not be possible within the agency in which they are employed, and in many cases would not meet the immediate, pressing needs of the patients for whom they are responsible. Thus, while concern for human rights, social justice and empowerment can be seen as integral to even highly bureaucratised social work roles, the wording of the IFSW definition, which appears to imply that social workers should be agitators for political change through their work, needs to be revised in favour of a version that acknowledges that social workers can often only operate at the micro level. The very real difference to individuals' lives that social workers can make should not be undervalued because they are not able to match a definition of their role that is not a true reflection of the realities of statutory social work with adults in the UK.

Notes

1 The HSW is implying that the patient will be unable to walk to the toilet on his own, and will therefore be forced to use incontinence pads.
2 A steady is a piece of equipment used to transfer patients from bed to the toilet or a chair. Again, the implication is that the patient will lose mobility.

7 The social work 'cuckoo' in the hospital 'nest'

Introduction

This chapter will explore the way the HSWs respond to and negotiate the working environment of the hospital and the patterns of their relationships with clinicians and ward managers. Drawing on the work of Irving Goffman, emphasis will be placed on the performative aspects of the HSWs' practices and the ways in which their presentation of a working self appears incongruous with many of the accepted forms of self-presentation common to clinicians. I will argue that this incongruity goes beyond conflicting expectations of role performance and is underpinned by fundamentally different conceptual 'frames' regarding the reality of work within the hospital. I will then turn attention to the ways in which HSWs manage their relationships with clinicians in order to ensure that they are able to contribute to the business of the hospital in a role that relies heavily on co-operation.

Goffman (1959) argued that human actions in the presence of others can be seen as performances in which the actor aims to project a version of her/himself that is germane to both the actor and the observer's shared understanding of the reality of the situation. All social activity is therefore guided by conscious and unconscious efforts to manage impressions and to negotiate identities. Typically, individuals in the presence of others deliberately seek to make their activity visible and comprehensible through visual signs and symbolic acts – to *dramatise* their actions in front of an audience. Impressions and identities are managed not only by individuals, but by teams of people with an interest in maintaining a common version of reality. In exploring the dramaturgical aspects of social interaction, therefore, the use of setting and props is of interest as well as the words and deeds of the actors. While Goffman's work has been criticised for focusing too much on appearances (Gouldner, 1970) and for reducing all human conduct to mere role-playing (MacIntyre, 1981) it provides a useful framework for analysing the strategic behaviours of people during interactions with others and the ways in which people conform to social norms (Burns, 1992). Goffman's contention is not that people spend their lives playing out parts insincerely, but that social action is orientated towards creating and maintaining shared meaning and shared interpretation.

A status, a position, a social place is not a material thing to be possessed and then displayed; it is a pattern of appropriate conduct, coherent, embellished and well-articulated.

(Goffman, 1959, p. 81)

Goffman's dramaturgical insights are complemented by his later work, *Frame Analysis* (Goffman, 1974), which seeks to answer William James's question, 'Under what circumstances do we think things are real?' (Burns, 1992, p. 247). Frames can be understood as being 'composed of little tacit theories about what exists, what happens and what matters' (Gitlin, 1980, p. 60). Framing therefore constitutes the meaning structure actors draw on to make sense of their situation and frames are shared by people interacting to guide their actions (Goffman, 1974). Thus, for example, a punch thrown by a player during a rugby match might be seen as no more than an act of foul play within the game, whereas a punch thrown within a pub or on the street would be likely to be treated as a criminal assault. Frames are continually renegotiated through interactions and are not reproduced perfectly, meaning that slippage can occur (Collins, 2004). Ambiguity may arise when actors do not share the same frame but neither is willing or able to adapt (Gray et al., 2015) – and this is often the case between the HSWs and the clinicians. In such circumstances, it is still possible for those interacting to work together, especially where there is a shared goal (Donnellon et al., 1986; Reay and Hinings, 2009).

The dramatisation and visibility of social work in the hospital

The self-presentation of HSWs was observed to be markedly different to that of clinicians within the hospital. An immediately visible difference noted during the fieldwork was that the HSWs do not wear uniforms, whereas all clinicians apart from doctors do. The uniforms worn by nurses, physiotherapists and occupational therapists all reflect the physical nature of their role – with nurses wearing overalls that are comfortable and cool, the colour of which indicates their level of responsibility and expertise, while occupational therapists and physiotherapists wear hospital-issued clothes that allow them to move freely and quickly should they need to provide physical support to patients, in the form of polo shirts, trainers and trousers of light and stretchy fabric. Although doctors are not required to wear uniform, their appearance nonetheless makes their role easily identifiable. Junior doctors are recognisable by a stethoscope worn around the neck over casual office clothes, while more senior doctors tend to wear office clothes that are more formal, yet with their pager prominently visible. Like the junior doctors, the HSWs wear smart casual office clothes, yet have no accoutrements to display their role or status, other than a diary, which is often stuffed full of pieces of paper and held shut with an elastic band. The lack of visual symbols of recognition for HSWs is significant because it reflects the low visibility of much of their work. I suggest that the low visibility and low-key dramatisation of social work within the hospital brings both benefits and challenges to the HSWs.

The low visibility of the social work team I observed was increased by the relative remoteness of their office.

> The building is in an isolated position some distance from the main hospital building and is shabby and uninviting from the outside. There is no sign indicating that this is where the team is based, and no obvious way for a visitor to gain entry, as the doors are secured with a combination lock.
>
> (Fieldnote)

Much of the daily activity of the HSWs takes place inside their offices, where they write up assessments and care plans, contact patients' relatives by telephone and make telephone calls to other professionals both within and outside the hospital. They do not carry pagers and often divert their desk phones to the team administrators' office in order to enable them to concentrate on writing up assessments that are required urgently. This means that it can be difficult for clinicians and ward managers to contact HSWs directly when they need to (although there is always an administrator able to take and pass on messages). Other professionals rarely visit the HSWs in their offices, which could therefore be considered a 'backstage' area for the performance of the social work role (Goffman, 1959). By contrast, the setting in which clinicians operate has a more complex 'frontstage/backstage' interplay (Lewin and Reeves, 2011), with much of the work of clinicians being visible to both patients and colleagues and therefore 'frontstage', yet with opportunities for 'backstage' work arising frequently through conversations in corridors and side offices. HSWs' lack of a continuous physical presence around the wards therefore not only obscures the performance of their role from clinical colleagues, but also excludes them from informal opportunities for building collegiate relationships.

A striking visual clue regarding the (in)visibility of the HSWs can be found by contrasting the physical presentation of the interior of their offices with presentations that are to be encountered elsewhere in the hospital. Goffman (1959) argues that the physical setting in which interactions occur is an integral part of the 'front' which performers create. The HSWs' offices give the impression of a team whose status is low and for whom keeping up appearances is of minor concern:

> Within [the HSWs' building], small offices run along a gloomy corridor. In one office, paint has peeled away from the wall and in general the offices are in a poor state of decoration, with furnishings that are old but functional. The building seems to get too cold in the winter and too hot in the summer. Even during bright days most of the offices require artificial lighting. Some social workers personalise their desk and working areas with photographs or pictures yet these scarcely diminish the overall impression of an unkempt, un-cared-for space. An unused office at the end of the corridor is used as a makeshift staff room and many of the

social workers use this to eat lunch together, often buying food from the hospital canteen to take back with them.

(Fieldnote)

The shabby appearance of the HSWs' office reflects its status as a 'backstage' area, which means, significantly, that it is also a setting which HSWs cannot use in managing impressions. By contrast, the office of the 'bedflow' managers, where a senior HSW has a daily meeting to discuss delays in patients' discharges (see Chapter 5) is a hive of technology and buzzing activity:

> The room is laid out with computers arranged in rows. The floor and walls are brightly clean and large windows look out over the city. All of the computer settings appear to be 'hot desks' and nobody leaves any personal touches. On one wall are two large flat screen televisions with information graphics related to the availability of beds or general messages for staff. The room is a hive of activity with bedflow managers to-ing and fro-ing. Some have telephone devices hanging from their necks by a cord, which they are able to speak into to dial numbers.

(Fieldnote)

The physical setting of the 'bedflow' managers' office gives a powerful representation of business, efficiency and command of the situation. It is in such an environment that the senior HSW must give a daily account of the work of the team, inevitably explaining delays. In the face of such a powerful dramatisation of the hospital's work, HSWs have limited resources to project an image of their work that reflects how they might wish to be seen.

Just as a contrast may be noted between the visual presentation of clinicians and HSWs, there appears to be a marked difference in the way HSWs and clinicians are able to dramatise their roles (Goffman, 1959). Many of the tasks performed by clinicians are easily intelligible to an observer: medical or surgical procedures are performed; equipment is used to monitor patients' vital functions; drugs are given; records are made in patients' charts, etc. By contrast, HSWs' actions with patients are less overtly dramatised, usually consisting only of a conversation with the patient in whatever location is most convenient for the patient. HSWs can make the accomplishment of their work known to clinicians by making recordings in medical notes, but cannot make the meaning of their interactions with patients known to clinicians purely through dramatic performance. Preservation of confidentiality means that HSWs tend to keep their interactions with patients as low-key as possible. By looking alone, one can tell whether a nurse is taking blood pressure or giving medication; by contrast, it is often not possible to tell by looking at a HSW in conversation with a patient whether she is a professional performing an assessment or a visitor discussing the weather.

The low visibility to clinicians of the HSWs' activities, and the difficulty the HSWs experience with dramatising their role, leads to misunderstandings and frustrations between them and the clinicians:

HSW9 says that some nurses think that they have to keep ringing up in order to prompt social workers to respond, and will ring several times a day. 'They don't seem to realise we have other cases.'

(Fieldnote)

HSW5 tells me that very often ward staff will claim that the social worker is delaying discharge when they are not... She speculates that sometimes nurses see that a referral has been made to social work and therefore automatically assume they are causing a delay.

(Fieldnote)

Because of the lack of visibility of social work, clinical staff on the wards appear to have little confidence in the ability or willingness of HSWs and therefore seek reassurance in a manner that can be experienced as mild harassment. The number of cases held by each HSW, the urgent demands that may be arising from other patients and the bureaucratic processes the HSWs must follow in order to obtain a service for patients (see Chapter 5) are not apparent to clinicians on each ward, to whom the HSW is an infrequent and fleeting visitor.

While it might be anticipated that promoting the visibility of their work might lead to more harmonious relations with clinicians and ward managers, in the dilemma of 'expression versus action' (Goffman, 1959, p. 42), the HSWs appear to have made a conscious choice to prioritise action over expression. This can be seen in the organisation of coverage of the hospital by the HSWs, and in their choice of which meetings they should attend. The HSWs are not allocated wards to cover, but range across the hospital according to the order in which patients are presented as cases for allocation. The result of this is that HSWs never work continuously on one particular ward for any length of time. This means that it is difficult for HSWs and clinicians to form close working relationships, since a HSW's time spent in any one ward will be limited and infrequent. Similarly, HSWs do not attend the weekly multi-disciplinary team meetings of any of the wards. While there would be too many wards for the HSWs to cover all, it might have been possible for them at least to attend the three rehabilitation wards, from which they frequently receive referrals. In the perception of HSWs, however, their more visible presence, either as a ward's allocated HSW or as a regular attendee at a multi-disciplinary meeting, would be likely to have an undesired effect:

HSW9 gets a call about a case that is not allocated to her. Afterwards she laughs and says that if you've been to a ward that day about one patient, if they have another who needs a social worker they'll invariably ring for you, as if you've suddenly become that ward's social worker. 'That can get really confusing when that patient isn't allocated to you.' HSW10 agrees, 'Yeah once a ward's seen you, they think you're theirs.' As they talk, exactly the same thing happens to HSW8, who comments, 'This is when it doesn't work so well, you see. You get pulled into things.'

(Fieldnote)

'Getting pulled into things' is seen as an undesirable distraction from the business of discharging patients. As was noted in the previous chapters, HSWs experience pressure from all sides to carry out discharges as quickly as possible and are also aware of the need to spread their resources as fairly and efficiently as possible for patients in need. While their lack of visibility causes some inconveniences in terms of their ability to communicate the nature of their daily work to clinicians, it also shields them from acquiring extra tasks outside the narrow bureaucratic functions that are their domain. As previously noted (see Craig and Muskat, 2013), there is a tendency for clinicians to look to HSWs to fulfil any miscellaneous tasks that do not touch on their own usual area of work. Maintaining a low level of visibility enables social workers to avoid such impositions and focus on the work that they identify as their own.

HSWs work in an environment in which multiple occupational groups stake claims for recognition through the dramatisation of their work, aided by their use of the setting and visual symbols of their roles. The HSWs' lack of control of a visible space within the setting, and the difficulty of dramatising their own role, might have been anticipated to be problematic for them in retaining any sense of autonomy or prestige. The HSWs turn their low visibility to their advantage, however, as a means of restricting the extent to which clinicians are able to make demands on their services.

Discrepant frames

The relatively low-key dramatisation of their work by HSWs is functional as a means of managing their workload, but may also serve another protective purpose. Despite the low levels of prestige enjoyed by social work in general as an occupation (see e.g. Judd and Sheffield, 2010), the HSWs in this study proved resistant to domination or control by doctors, in contrast to the other occupations involved with the care of patients observed. Indeed, in terms of Goffman's (1974) theory of frame analysis, it can be argued that the HSWs rely on a framing of inter-professional relations that is fundamentally different to that shared by clinicians. Their low-key dramatisation of their work might therefore be interpreted as a deliberate strategy to avoid overly frequent incidents of overt conflict with clinical colleagues. Rather than engage in such conflicts, HSWs pursue their work as they see fit to do it without drawing attention to fundamental disagreements with their clinical colleagues.

The frame shared by clinicians revolves around the doctor as the co-ordinator and overseer of each patient's care (Willis, 1989). While a hierarchy of authority exists, the social order of hospital teams is a negotiated one, since experienced practitioners in the lower ranking occupation of nursing may nonetheless demonstrate more power than junior doctors in the early stages of their career (Strauss et al., 1963). As other clinical occupations have emerged, such as physiotherapy and occupational therapy, the need has arisen for those practitioners to negotiate their own jurisdictions, the boundaries of which can be dynamic and contested (Abbott, 1988). The idea of a negotiated order implies active discussion of roles and duties, yet this does not always occur – often roles are agreed through tacit understandings (Allen, 1997). However power is distributed, and however collaboratively multi-disciplinary teams may work, it remains the case that authority over inpatient care ulti-mately lies with a doctor (Nugus et al., 2010). Clinical teams are not always ordered with the priorities of the patient at their centre – wards, units and speciality teams employ idiosyncratic logics that work to promote the inter-ests of clinicians in the organisation of their work (White et al., 2012).

During the fieldwork, it was possible to see the shared frame of clinicians at play in the rehabilitation hospital. The weekly multi-disciplinary team (MDT) meetings of two wards were observed on multiple occasions. Notable in both were the extent to which the most senior doctor controlled the conduct of the meeting, deciding when it was time to move the discussion on and inviting other clinicians in turn to make their reports. The more senior the doctor who chaired the meeting, the more structured the meeting was. HSWs were nota-ble for their absence from these meetings, which was sometimes remarked on by clinicians discussing the social needs of patients. We might interpret the MDT meeting as a team performance that reinforces the social order (Goff-man, 1959), and if so, then the HSWs' absence from it appears to be an act of non-conformity to that order and to the shared frame that underpins it.

In contrast to the frame held by clinicians, the frame shared in common by the HSWs emphasises the HSW's obligation to the bureaucratic structures that govern their work (see previous chapter) and their independence from the clinical team in decision-making. Both of these assertions may be overlooked by clinicians:

> HSW10: Sometimes the OTs think that if they recommend, say, four calls, they think that's what it is, and that's what they tell families. They don't realise that I have to come in behind them and make my own assessment.
>
> (Fieldnote)

While the occupational therapist (OT) may make a recommendation about the nature of a care package that should be supplied by social services, the HSW must make her own assessment, in which the OT's recommendation is one of many pieces of information to be taken into consideration. Also to be considered are the patient's wishes, the capabilities and willingness of informal carers to provide assistance and the information provided by other clinicians. The HSW must then match this information against the eligibility criteria used by the local authority to supply services. That OTs fail to recognise the independence of HSWs in acting on their recommendations suggests that this may be an area of occupational boundary disputes (Abbott, 1988), albeit one in which, for the time being, HSWs have the upper hand. It is also indicative of a lack of a shared understanding of roles and expectations.

Clinicians' recognition of the authority of HSWs to make independent decisions is undermined by the reliance of HSWs on the information provided by clinicians, which results in doubts about HSWs' knowledge claims:

> It's not just me – lots of OTs feel that social workers just use their assessments rather than doing any real work themselves.
>
> (Interview – OT2)

> I can't even say they've got the knowledge of the care package, because in health, if we do continuing healthcare, we do the care plans, and know what package of care. They're very much guided by health, aren't they, on what people can do, their medical knowledge isn't as great as ours, so they might get a diagnosis but they're not really that familiar with it, because we put in a lot of continuing healthcare applications and they're not that familiar with what the medical terms are.
>
> (Interview – Ward Sister 1)

The overlap of knowledge and roles between OTs, nurses and HSWs weakens the HSWs' claim to have a unique set of competencies that might command respect within the hospital hierarchy. HSWs are seen by their clinician colleagues to collect information, but the work that they do in co-ordinating the information and weighing it up against other information that they have collected for themselves is largely invisible. The frame in which HSWs see themselves as independent decision-makers is therefore unknown to clinicians.

While the frame of HSWs is unfamiliar to many clinicians, HSWs are familiar with the clinicians' frame. The HSWs' frame is not one in which the hierarchy of professional authority and knowledge claims is unacknowledged, but rather one in which it is irrelevant. The HSWs do demonstrate consciousness that the knowledge claims of doctors are superior to their own, e.g.:

> HSW10: It's hard because we don't have their knowledge, we can just say what the patient is telling us.
>
> (Fieldnote)

Further, when speaking to doctors during formal meetings HSWs tend to use a studied politeness, for example addressing them as, 'Doctor'. Thus, HSWs show a working knowledge of the frame shared by clinicians, even if they do not share it. Despite the respect accorded to doctors, however, HSWs retain a strong sense of independence from the hospital hierarchy. Their assertion of independence from the hierarchy is linked to their positioning as advocates for patients. As the manager of the team put it during a team meeting,

It's our job to be advocating for patients.

(Fieldnote)

The meaning of advocacy in terms of what HSWs seek to accomplish for patients was explored in Chapter 6. Of note here is that the positioning of the HSWs as advocates means that HSWs do not feel obliged to observe the usual proprieties that come from partaking in a team performance, such as hiding disagreement from outsiders and deferring decisions to those with claims to higher authority (Goffman, 1959). Their independence means that they are able to define what their role is and what it is not, and therefore to retain some control over the nature of their work.

On both sides, the discrepant frames can be a source of frustration. Doctors, for example, may resent the fact that they are not able to direct HSWs' activities in order to relieve themselves of the need to deal with the social aspects of patients' needs:

> The doctor says that he is having to do things that really aren't in his remit and that he ought to be freed up to get on with his medical duties by having social workers to deal with the other problems.
>
> (Fieldnote – conversation between Dr 2 and Ward Sister 2)

Doctors tend to seek to restrict their work to the performance of clinical competencies and seek to distribute tasks that do not provide the opportunity for clinical performance elsewhere (Latimer, 2000). In this doctor's view, the HSWs should be available as a resource to do just this, but the HSWs' elusiveness and independence from the hierarchy means that this is not possible. Whereas the HSWs are aware of the clinicians' framing of the social order of the hospital, but understand themselves as operating outside it, clinicians show little awareness of HSWs' different frame. HSWs' failure to practice as doctors wish they would is therefore experienced by clinicians as a violation of the hospital's social order.

The HSWs are aware of the frustrations of clinicians, but frame the issue as a misunderstanding of their role, rather than a failing on their part:

> [T]they don't understand our processes. I think if they understood what we have to go through to get a package of care, or to enable to us to go forward with a placement, they may be a little bit more sympathetic. But they don't, they don't understand what we do …
>
> (Interview – HSW1)

There is a clear sense of alienation between the social workers and the clinicians. It is interesting that the HSW places emphasis on the bureaucratic function as the unique aspect of social work that is not understood by her colleagues in health care. This highlights the contrast between social work's frame, which is orientated around the local authority's bureaucratic functions in which procedure is central, and the frame of clinicians within the hospital, whose work must often be accomplished as a response to immediate and pressing need, and is therefore less constrained by process and authorisation (Allen, 1997). The HSWs' position outside the hospital hierarchy should not be understood as a sign of their autonomy, since they have obligations, which are no less binding, to the bureaucratic order through which their work must be processed.

Operating with frame discrepancy within the hospital is not a comfortable experience for the HSWs, particularly because their work relies on good communication with their clinical colleagues. As noted in Chapter 5, completing assessments is the central task of the HSWs' role, and is one in which HSWs must rely heavily on the information provided by clinicians. HSWs are sensitive to the inconvenience providing such information can cause clinicians:

> I think they probably see me as being a pain, more than anything. Because I think they probably think, 'Oh no, social worker's requested this, social worker's requested that.' So I think sometimes they may see me as a barrier to actually discharging someone.
>
> (Interview – HSW4)

The information the HSWs receive from clinicians is often incomplete, meaning that HSWs are obliged to chase clinicians in order to complete their assessments. The anxiety this can cause to HSWs reflects their position as an outsider in the hospital setting, and an outsider to clinical ways of working, which tend to focus on the immediate needs of the body (Allen, 1997). The position of outsider for HSWs is reinforced by the fact that they are employees of a separate agency, which means that the communication of changing policies and priorities on either side is minimal.

The disparate frames of the HSWs and clinicians and the outsider position of the HSWs can give rise to a mutual mistrust, which can be seen to manifest itself in tales that are told on both sides about the nefariousness of the others' practices. The tales told by clinicians and social workers about each other bear a remarkable similarity:

> I went up to another hospital once for this one lady. I started to do a full UAP [Unified Assessment Process] for her but quickly realised she had lots of fast-track CHC [Continuing Healthcare] triggers. I pointed this out to health, and apparently someone had told them that the patient would get services faster through social services. But legally, it had to be CHC because it was nursing care. She was on so much morphine she didn't know who she was.
>
> (Fieldnote – HSW10)

The ward sister says that she believes that social workers use the CHC process to delay the need to do a social work assessment. She cites a recent case where everyone involved in the meeting except the social worker felt that the needs were not CHC, but the social worker felt that it was, so the application was put forward and then 'thrown back.' The ward sister thinks it should be documented in the process as to who agrees and disagrees with the application.

(Fieldnote from ward visit)

In both passages quoted, there is the belief that professionals are trying to 'cheat' the system, whether to obtain priority for a patient or to avoid the necessity of more in-depth work. The practice of privately accusing the other side of unfair practices is a means by which individuals within a team bond and can also be a way of fostering a shared sense of professional identity (Dingwall, 1977). Common to both passages, however, is misunderstanding that arises from disparate frames. In the first passage, clinicians mistakenly assume that HSWs will do whatever is quickest and most expedient for the immediate needs of the patient, rather than observing the proper bureaucratic protocols to which they are obliged to adhere. In the second passage, the ward sister's belief that the social workers push for CHC to avoid extra work is probably unfounded, since the HSWs claim that a similar amount of work is required from them whether a patient is to receive CHC or local authority-funded care. The HSW's position in pushing for the CHC application to go ahead therefore is most likely to arise from acting as a patient's advocate (CHC funding provided by the NHS is desirable for patients and carers because it is not means-tested, unlike the care packages provided by local authorities.) The ward sister's interpretation of HSWs' motives therefore overlooks the importance of patient advocacy within the HSW role and the deliberate positioning of HSWs on the side of patients.

HSWs appear to work within a frame that can be distinguished from that of the clinicians. Whereas clinicians embrace a complex social order involving negotiation and hierarchy, with a senior doctor retaining oversight and final say over patient care, the HSWs retain a sense of independence from the hospital order and a loyalty to their agency's bureaucratic order. Clinicians are often unaware of the disparate frame through which the HSWs view their work, yet HSWs are aware of the clinicians' frame, even though they do not accept its relevance to them. Both of these frames represent reality as understood by those who hold them (Goffman, 1974) and therefore guide their actions and expectations.

Frame conflicts

It is striking that, though HSWs often show awareness of the clinicians' frame, they do not readily adapt themselves to it. Goffman (1981, p. 156) argued that nimble social actors are able to switch 'footing' – meaning that they are able to change the alignment of their behaviour to match the frames of others with whom they are interacting. Tannen and Wallat (1987) give the example of a paediatrician modulating her language and gestures during a consultation depending on whether she was talking to a child, the child's mother or to medical students. The HSWs' positioning as advocates for patients, however, means that the assumption of a subordinate position, by adopting the footing of the clinicians' frame, is not an option. While the low-key dramatisation of HSWs' work may minimise conflict with clinicians over their role and practices, some incidences of open conflict arising from frame differences are therefore inevitable. An example of overt conflict occurred during an assessment meeting for a patient's CHC application:

> Dr 4 emphasises he does not think the application has any chance of success with the panel and therefore feels it should not go ahead. HSW5 asks aren't all his needs in the nature of his illness? Dr 4 says insistently that he is a Parkinson's specialist and he would say he is in a complex stage but he does not need extraordinary nursing care. HSW5 questions this – the illness is causing his nursing care needs. She turns to the family and asks them if they want to apply. The doctor says he does not want to waste time.
>
> (Fieldnote)

The HSW's positioning as an advocate for the patient allows her to challenge the doctor's opinions in front of the patient's relatives, an action that would usually be regarded as taboo by other members of a team (Goffman, 1959). The HSW's questioning of the doctor's opinion causes him discomfiture and prompts him to make an open claim to superior knowledge, as an assertion of his place high in the hierarchy of authority. The HSW's response is equally assertive in its way – by turning to the family members representing the patient in the meeting and asking them if they want to go ahead with the application anyway, she displays that the hierarchy is of no consequence to her, since the nature of her role is so different to that of clinicians. Thus, two different frames are brought into open conflict. In the doctor's frame, his opinion on the matter is final and, as a subordinate member of the team, the HSW must accept it. In her frame, the HSW places herself outside the doctor's authority, as the patient's advocate, and thus is able to challenge him.

The conflict, on this occasion, was resolved by the HSW temporarily deferring to the doctor's opinion. The challenge was not sustained and the meeting ended with an agreement that the patient's application would not succeed, and therefore would not be taken forward. After the meeting had formally finished, both the HSW and senior nurse stayed with the patient's relatives to soothe their disappointment and answer any further questions they might have. The senior nurse then left, yet the HSW remained with the relatives and, in privacy, offered some advice to them:

> As soon as the nurse is gone, HSW5 advises the family members to wait and get a new CHC assessment once patient is in the community. She says the community nurses are much more thorough and more likely to get the sort of detail needed to get this through.
>
> (Fieldnote)

While the HSW did not pursue open conflict with the doctor further than an initial questioning of his opinion, nor did she concede the matter entirely. She instead chose actions that were invisible to the clinicians, but which remained effective for her purpose of ensuring that the patient might access CHC funding if at all possible. Thus, the HSW made a pragmatic decision that it was not possible to persuade the doctor, but did not bend herself entirely to the hospital frame in which the doctor's say is final.

Situations do sometimes arise in which HSWs do not back down from conflict. Another HSW returning to the office from a CHC meeting described what transpired when, at the end of the meeting he refused to withdraw his disagreement with the doctor over a patient's application:

> She [the chair of the meeting] kept saying to me, 'We're in dispute.' I said, 'Well I'm not in dispute, I just have a different view.' But she kept coming back to this, saying, 'We're in dispute,' as if it was something very dramatic. So I said, 'Well what does that mean?' And it just means that all the paperwork gets sent up to the next level for a decision. Well, I don't mind. If the decision goes against me, so be it. It's up to the family to appeal. I'm not going to get excited about it. Not as excited as the chair was anyway.
>
> (Fieldnote – HSW3)

In order for a CHC application to progress or to be dismissed, there needs to be agreement between representatives of both the NHS and local authority. That disagreements rarely happen can be inferred from the way the HSW described the chair presenting being 'in dispute' in a dramatic fashion. This also suggests that the HSW's words were in violation of the usual social order of the hospital, again arising from disparate frames. The HSWs' frame is one in which conflict with clinicians is a necessary part of the job, whereas, within the clinicians' frame, the hierarchical social order prevents conflict.

Disputes within CHC assessment have a formal arrangement for resolution, involving referral to managers on both sides at a higher level. Where such mechanisms are not in place, however, disputes between HSWs and clinicians can lead to an impasse:

> There was a gentleman, from the first day I met him, I felt he didn't have capacity with regards to discharge destination because he couldn't retain information, he wasn't able to weigh up any risks, and we did a risk assessment with him, and his responses were just completely inappropriate, whereas the doctor thought that he had capacity. I challenged him on this and his response was, 'Oh, HSW1 [he called her by her first name], I have no doubt in my mind that he has capacity.' And I said, 'Well I'm sorry but, you know, I disagree. I'll come back and visit him in a few days.' I went back, I was still adamant he didn't have capacity. The doctor was adamant that he did, and the gentleman started deteriorating.

And it took about six weeks and the doctor actually said, 'He doesn't have capacity.' Whereas this gentleman has gone from residential to needing a nursing home and now CHC. And the family had actually chosen a residential home that they thought their father would have been happy in, but now he couldn't go.

(Interview – HSW1)

Conflict without arbitration in this example led to an impasse that proved harmful to the patient. Under the Mental Capacity Act 2005, decisions can be made on behalf of a person who is deemed to lack capacity to make their own decisions. Because there were two competing capacity assessments, however, no action could be taken for the patient until the disagreement was resolved. In this case, while the doctor eventually moved to the HSW's position, this might have been in response to the changing presentation of the patient rather than a deliberate decision to acquiesce to the HSW's point of view. As noted in the previous chapters, HSWs usually rely on doctors to make capacity assessments. This HSW's willingness to challenge a doctor's assessment reinforces the suggestion made in Chapter 5 that HSWs' reliance on doctors for capacity assessment arises from convenience rather than deference to doctors' expertise. The HSWs' recognition of the superior knowledge claims of doctors as professionals therefore does not extend beyond the doctor's area of medical expertise. While, in his frame, the senior doctor may expect all clinical opinions he gives to be deferred to as a matter of course, the HSWs operate in a frame in which doctors' opinions outside their medical speciality cannot claim higher rank.

The HSW went on to describe further disagreement with this doctor during the subsequent CHC meeting for the same patient:

I challenged him on one of the domains, and his response was, 'We need to get somebody more senior than yourself to attend the meeting.'

(Interview – HSW1)

The doctor's request for a more senior social worker to attend the meeting represents an attack on the legitimacy of the HSW's role performance (Goffman, 1959). It might also be interpreted as a further example of frame conflict. The senior doctor's place near the top of the hierarchy within the hospital relies on his having the highest knowledge claim and certified credentials (Macdonald, 1995). His request for a more senior HSW would appear to imply that this HSW's experience and knowledge is insufficient to understand the issues or to challenge his opinion. By contrast, the HSW frame places far less emphasis on experience and credentials in the distribution of work and responsibilities. Traditionally, within the occupation of social work in general, while obviously complex cases would be reserved for the most experienced practitioners, there was comparatively little distinction in terms of career progression and grading between practitioners of vast experience and practitioners who were new to the role (Munro, 2011). While the picture has changed a little with the introduction of 'consultant social worker' and 'principal officer' posts in many local authorities, the structure of this particular hospital social work team still runs along the traditional lines. The duties of a HSW in this team therefore mean that even an inexperienced practitioner might be expected to challenge the opinion of a senior doctor.

Frame conflicts appear to arise because the frame of HSWs is not recognised by clinicians, and because HSWs resist the clinicians' frame. Clinicians often expect HSWs to operate within the clinicians' frame and the hierarchical order that is central to it. The HSWs' frame is underpinned by their self-definition as advocates for patients and a loyalty to their own bureaucratic order rather than the social order of the clinicians. HSWs' positioning as patient advocates enables them to be resilient against the claims of the clinicians' frame, because the role of an advocate implies willingness to stand in opposition when necessary.

Maintaining harmony

This chapter has so far focused on the ways in which HSWs and clinicians view the world differently, and the overt conflicts which can arise as a result. It would be misleading, however, to understand the hospital as a place of continual conflict and misunderstanding between HSWs and clinicians. Most of the time, all HSWs are able to form and maintain positive and harmonious working relationships with clinicians. Doing so involves a deliberate projection of self on the part of HSWs:

> [I]nitially you need to be very sociable I would say with everybody... you need to get on well and build up that rapport with people because that tends to be how you get the best results then, you know, being able to both work together towards the goal of getting somebody home.
>
> (Interview – HSW10)

HSWs may go for several months without involvement with a given ward, meaning that it is difficult for HSWs and clinicians to share any sense of continuity in their working relationships. Furthermore, the nurses, whose information is so important to the social work assessment, work irregular shift patterns, which means that social workers will often have to speak to several different nurses on one-off occasions during the course of working with just one patient. Thus, HSWs will often have to ask people with whom they are not very familiar to complete paperwork for them. The sociable demeanour which HSWs therefore have to project when dealing with clinicians is a form of emotional labour (Hochschild, 2012), without which the HSWs would struggle to accomplish their work. The extent to which their sociable displays are purely external 'surface acting' or more internalised 'deep acting' (Grandey, 2003) varies between individuals, yet all HSWs are obliged to maintain a sociable front in order to negotiate the work with clinicians.

While personal friendliness is obligatory for HSWs in their dealings with clinicians, collaborative work is made possible when practitioners with different perspectives share a sense of purpose and a common goal (Reay and Hinings, 2009). Central to the successful co-operation between HSWs and clinicians, therefore, is the shared sense of doing the best for the patient. The low level of dramatisation of their work by HSWs, while it has its advantages, means that the ways through which HSWs contribute to the shared aim of 'what is best for the patient' are sometimes obscured. Speaking about a complex discharge that had gone well, one HSW described the change in clinicians' attitudes brought about by a better understanding of the patient's issues:

> In the beginning, they just wanted her out, because they weren't aware of all the POVA [protection of vulnerable adults] issues and the on-going issues, but then when they did witness a few things on the ward, they were quite supportive as well, because we had the discharge liaison nurse attending meetings with me, so that I had people from health and social services that were on the same hymn sheet. And, towards the end, they were very supportive, they weren't happy with the length of stay in the hospital but I actually had a thank you off the senior nurse for the discharge – and a hug off the doctor ...
>
> (Interview – HSW1)

It is significant that the HSW cited ward staff directly witnessing some of the safeguarding issues as a key turning point, highlighting the advantages visibility of work may bring for HSWs in their relationships with clinicians. Where clinicians are able to see that HSWs' work is congruent with their understanding of what is best for the patient, they are more likely to be supportive and tolerant. The same is true of HSWs' attitude to clinicians.

Just as a sense of shared purpose can unite HSWs and clinicians, a common enemy can have a similar effect. Facing adversity together can often enable people operating with discordant frames to bond (Reay and Hinings, 2005). The fact that HSWs and clinicians work for different agencies means that shared experience of adversity in terms of organisational threats such as redundancies or changes to working conditions is not available. Where patients or their relatives present a threat, however, whether physical or in terms of potential litigation, HSWs and clinicians tend to close ranks. For example, one HSW described being supported by a nursing manager to leave a meeting when a patient's relative became verbally abusive. The same HSW also recounted the story of a time she took herself to stand physically close to a nurse who clearly felt threatened by a patient's relative who was shouting at her in the middle of a ward. Similarly, HSWs who had been involved with patients whose issues were likely to be brought before the Court of Protection[1] described feeling supported by their clinical colleagues. Social workers also actively seek the support of clinical colleagues when faced with adverse reactions from patients or carers. For example, during the fieldwork, one HSW was called upon to deal with a telephone call from a carer whom she described as 'abusive'.

After the telephone call, one of the other social workers goes to admin worker 2 (who fielded the call first) to check that she is alright and offer her some comfort. The social worker advises the admin worker just to take a message for HSW2 to call the carer back next time. Nobody checks if HSW2 is alright. HSW2 goes back to her office and immediately telephones the ward where the patient concerned is, and relates the story of the telephone call she just had, placing emphasis on the carer's abusiveness and bad language.

(Fieldnote)

It is interesting that the other HSWs did not feel the need to comfort HSW2 or see to her welfare, the assumption being that dealing with angry or abusive people is part of the social work role. HSW2's telephone call to the ward therefore represents behaviour aimed at seeking validation and closeness from the clinicians. This illustrates how social workers actively employ strategies to build personal connections with clinicians to help them to deal with the challenges arising in their work.

Maintaining a working relationship with clinicians can be challenging when HSWs take decisions that go against clinicians' wishes. Sometimes overt conflict can be averted by HSWs' presentation of a sociable front. For example, one HSW came across a patient who had been told by ward staff that he would be discharged that day, which was impossible because he had not had time to arrange the care he would need at home. While this caused anger to the HSW, which was expressed in the 'backstage' area of the HSWs' offices, he used humour when dealing directly with ward staff:

I rang the ward and said, 'Do I need to put my armour on when I come up?' They said, 'We're not like that.'

(Fieldnote – HSW4)

The HSW was aware that blocking the patient's discharge would cause difficulties for the ward, since it would mean having to rearrange the planned care for other patients and would involve discussion with the hospital's patient flow managers. Expecting hostility when he went to the ward, he therefore rang ahead to diffuse the tension. Making a joke about the disagreement over the patient's care represents an instance of role distance, in which a person distances her/himself from the role being performed (Goffman, 1961). By stressing his vulnerability when entering a potentially hostile ward, the HSW sought to separate the ward clinicians' perception of his self from the role he was performing. He later confirmed that he had been able to retain a friendly working relationship with the clinicians involved, suggesting that the ploy was successful.

HSWs actively strive to maintain harmonious working relationships with colleagues, despite their differing frames. Where possible, they play down the significance of conflict and foster a sense of collegiality, particularly through uniting against adversity. Common to both clinicians and HSWs is an avowed commitment to doing their best for the patient. This provides a shared sense of purpose which overrides tensions and conflicts between the HSWs and clinicians for most of the time.

Conclusion

This chapter has examined the self-presentation of HSWs and the framing through which they understand their world of work. In contrast to the frame shared by clinicians, which emphasises the authority of doctors in making decisions over patient care, HSWs see themselves as independent decision-makers who operate outside the hierarchical order of clinicians, owing loyalty instead to their agency's bureaucratic order. The low-level dramatisation of their work assists the HSWs in retaining their independence from the clinicians' hierarchy, yet some conflicts are inevitable. Where significant conflicts occur, the discrepancy of framing is often apparent. Despite these differences, relationships between HSWs and clinicians are usually harmonious. HSWs' interactions with clinicians are orientated towards establishing and maintaining collaborative relationships, and deliberate strategies are sometimes employed for this end.

Note

1 The Court of Protection makes decisions on financial or welfare matters for people who are deemed to lack mental capacity to make such decisions for themselves at the time the decision needs to be made.

8 Conclusions

Summary of research findings

Exploration of the ethnographic findings of my study began in Chapter 5 with an examination of the tasks that hospital social workers (HSWs) carry out, the influence of managerial techniques on their practices and the dehumanising nature of the bureaucratic system in which they work. The focus of the work of HSWs is on arranging the discharges of patients from hospital beds once they are considered medically fit by clinicians, either by arranging a package of community care or arranging for the patient to go into residential care. A sense of pressure on the HSWs to accomplish each discharge as quickly as possible is maintained by hospital managers and clinicians, supported by senior managers within the HSWs' employing local authority. The new public management technique of measuring quantitative performance indicators is used by managers in both the NHS and local authority as a tool for maintaining this pressure and monitoring the HSWs' performance. While this technique can be effective for the managers in identifying particular instances of delay and requiring HSWs to address them immediately, it does not have the effect of focusing HSWs solely on the speediest discharge for each patient. HSWs' concerns do not lie solely with serving the system as efficiently as possible because they do not have a personal stake in the performance data (i.e. they are not directly rewarded if their data are deemed good). The well-being of the patient and carers therefore remains of greater to concern to HSWs than being seen to work efficiently and HSWs effectively strive to strike a balance between the two.

Despite HSWs' willingness to balance the need to work efficiently with a concern for ensuring that the best interests of the patient are served, it is possible to detect the dehumanising effects of bureaucracy in their work. Fordist and Taylorist techniques are used to ensure that HSWs perform their tasks as quickly and efficiently as possible (Dustin, 2007). These limit the extent to which HSWs are able to be involved in the wider emotional or social world of the patient. The system of authorisation for the care plans proposed by HSWs (which is common throughout UK community care) means that managers who are never in direct contact with the people affected can refuse the services HSWs deem them to need. Thus, the social work bureaucracy separates the decision-maker from witnessing the consequences of her/his decision and therefore removes some of the moral dimensions of the decision, which becomes one of eligibility and resource availability only (Bauman, 1989). The system in which HSWs operate requires that they undertake some highly rationalised and dehumanising tasks, such as assessment of patients for NHS Continuing Healthcare funding. Rationalisation of their tasks is functional for the HSWs in spreading their limited resources as fairly and efficiently as possible, however. Even in the context of a highly bureaucratised role, the concept of street level bureaucracy (Lipsky, 1980) remains relevant. HSWs retain a certain level of discretion, which they sometimes use to bring about a favourable outcome for a patient or to seek time to make a fuller exploration of a patient's circumstances. On other occasions, however, their discretion is used to enable them to make their work less complicated and to protect themselves from taking on further responsibilities, as suggested by Lipsky (1980).

The heavily bureaucratised nature of hospital social work as described in Chapter 5 might cause the reader to ask whether this work is really social work at all. Chapter 6 therefore explored the extent to which the practices of the HSWs in this study can be defined as 'social work'. A working description of social work was adapted from the IFSW (2014) definition, through which it was argued that regard for human rights, social justice and empowerment are central to any conception of social work. It was possible to trace the working of each of these values in the practices of the HSWs in this study, yet it was equally clear that the HSWs only put these values into operation at the interpersonal level, and that it would not be possible for them to agitate for wider social changes as a part of their everyday employment. With human rights, the HSWs prioritise negative rights that emphasise the freedom of the individual from interference by external forces; with social justice, the HSWs emphasise the welfare of the individual in isolation from the wider political context in which their need arises; and with empowerment, HSWs are only able to support the power of individuals to advance their own interests, without opportunities to connect individuals to more collective forms of power. Thus, the work of the HSWs might be defined as a liberal, rather than radical practice, which draws on a critical understanding of power, oppression and disadvantage, yet without advocating for solutions that address these directly. The radical social work critique might argue that this form of social work offers salve for some of the symptoms that oppression and disadvantage bring about, without addressing the underlying cause (Brake and Bailey, 1975). The potential of this type of work to cause material change for the better in the lives of people should not be underestimated, however, nor should the potential of social work to make structural changes be overestimated.

Within the liberal form of social work practised by the HSWs, it was clear that the principle of self-determination is the foundational value. The right of people to make their own decision about what happens to them was noted to be considered by HSWs to be a deontological imperative and a universal good. While human rights laws were not used by the HSWs as a means of defending people's self-determination, the denial of a patient's self-determination could only follow an assessment that s/he lacked capacity according to legally defined procedures and prescriptions. Thus, the HSWs consider self-determination to be a natural right, applicable to everyone in all but exceptional circumstances, rather than one that must be gifted through legislation. The HSWs promote patients' self-determination through their role in making care plans that put the wishes and choices of patients at their centre, and through the activity of advocacy. HSWs were noted to advocate on behalf of patients and carers to other professionals within the hospital, and to carers or family members who may have a different view to the patient about what the long-term plan should be. The discourse of risk might be used by HSWs either to promote positive risk-taking for patients for whom the benefits of a decision might outweigh the negatives (Morgan, 1996) or to prevent wards from discharging patients before it was physically safe for them to do so. Evidence from patients and carers gathered through the fieldwork would suggest that the HSWs' advocacy role is particularly valued by them. Limitations to HSWs' provision of advocacy were noted, however, revolving around their reluctance or perceived inability to challenge poor service provision by hospitals or care homes through raising concerns at a higher level.

Having explored the nature of the work in hospital social work, for the final empirical chapter, I turned attention to the self-presentation of HSWs and the way their work fits into the wider hospital setting. It was first noted that the self-presentation of HSWs as working professionals within the hospital is less visually and dramatically overt than that of clinicians. HSWs lack visual symbols of their working identity, have little command of the physical spaces of the hospital outside their offices (which, in the case of this team are geographically isolated from their clinical colleagues), and adopt a low-key dramatisation of their direct work with patients and carers, which is appropriate to the confidential work they must carry out. Far from indicating an occupational grouping that is lacking in self-confidence or subservient to the demands of clinicians, the low-key self-presentation of the HSWs is functional in allowing them to avoid extra demands on their services from clinicians, thus protecting the manageability of their workloads, and in enabling them to avoid domination or control by doctors. The independence of HSWs from the oversight of doctors is rooted in the HSWs' employment by a separate agency, yet is also maintained by deliberate strategic actions on the part of the HSWs.

Drawing on Goffman's theory of frame analysis (Goffman, 1974), I argued that the repeated assertion of their independence by the HSWs and the occasional mutual irritation between clinicians and HSWs reflect a discrepancy between the frames each grouping uses to make sense of the social world of the working hospital. The frame shared by clinicians generally positions the most senior doctor involved in a patient's care as having authority over all other professionals involved. By contrast, the HSWs consider themselves to sit outside of the clinicians' hierarchy and therefore regard the opinions of all doctors as only advisory for social work purposes. HSWs therefore are willing to challenge a senior doctor, even in front of the patient or carers, an action that would be socially unacceptable within the clinical team. In the matter of assessing patients' mental capacity, though HSWs often find it convenient to accept the assessments of doctors, they are willing to express a different opinion to the doctor if they decide that it is necessary to do so. Frustrations arise between the clinicians and the HSWs because the clinicians do not understand that the HSWs have a different frame to them and do not recognise the right of HSWs to operate outside the hierarchy that is central to the clinical frame. HSWs are aware of the frame discrepancy and can find the experience of working in the hospital uncomfortable at times. They therefore employ strategies to minimise conflict with their clinical colleagues, including cultivating a sociable demeanour, the use of humour, emphasising shared values and aims, and uniting when patients or their relatives show hostility. HSWs draw on their self-professed position as advocates for patients or carers to maintain their independence from the clinical frame and are resilient against becoming subordinate.

Hospital social work and liquid modernity

The empirical research discussed in this book has produced three clear messages about hospital social work:

1   The tasks performed by HSWs are shaped by bureaucracy and the neo-liberal model of state services, with an emphasis on the state purchasing services from private providers.
2   The HSWs work towards promoting patients' self-determination, social justice and empowerment at the individual level without engaging in any efforts to address wider social structures.
3   The HSWs deliberately maintain a distinct professional identity within the hospital.

Regarding points one and two, it would be all too easy to side with the pessimistic tone of much recent scholarship regarding social work with older people, lamenting the 'straitjacket' of community care (Lymbery, 2010), the McDonaldisation of social work (Dustin, 2007) and the loss of relational work (Sullivan, 2009). HSWs maintain a distinctive professional identity within the hospital for a reason that goes beyond loyalty to their bureaucracy, however. Their work with patients focuses on promoting individual rights that might otherwise be lost within the workings of the hospital and its clinicians. I argue, therefore, that social work has been developing, possibly unconsciously, a flexible response to the complexities of social life in the twenty-first century.

As noted in Chapter 1, Bauman's (2000a) concept of liquid modernity has relevance to the people with whom HSWs are concerned and their needs. Old age can be said to be 'liquid' with regards to the uncertainties that arise from chronic and progressive physical and mental illnesses that people of advancing years tend to encounter. With rising life expectancy, many older people are living for long periods in a state of increasing frailty and declining physical and mental health (Age UK, 2017). The course of the diseases of old age, such as dementia, Parkinson's Disease, cardiovascular illness and even some cancers, is predominantly progressive, yet progress is unpredictable for each individual (Barry and Yuill, 2016). Medical advances add to the uncertainty by prolonging life and offering hope of delaying disease progression. The liquid modern era, with its emphasis on individual choice and individual responsibility, thrusts on older people responsibility for coping alone with adverse health developments in their lives, yet, as Bauman notes, individuals are often 'equipped with tools and resources that are blatantly inadequate to the task' (Bauman, 2007, p. 14). The responsibility of older people as individuals to find their own ways of coping with age-related difficulties is underpinned by the dominance of neoliberalism in liquid modern societies, which produces welfare states that are only prepared to provide minimal services, yet equally makes it difficult for people of working age to take on caring responsibilities for their elderly relatives, since they are required to be available and flexible within the labour market.

In addition to the risk of facing the uncertainties arising from declining physical and mental health alone and ill-equipped, older people often also face a reduced ability to participate in the benefits of the liquid modern era. While the individual responsibility of the liquid modern era can be experienced as an inescapable fate (Bauman, 2000a), it can also be experienced as a liberating opportunity to engage in life politics and seek fulfilment through personal development (Giddens, 1992; 1999). Increasing mental and physical infirmity, however, may limit the liberty of older people to participate in life politics and cut off the succession of personal projects that often comprises the progression of the individual through life in liquid modernity (Bauman, 2000a). In responding to the needs of older people as they encounter them, HSWs are therefore responding to some of the dilemmas of liquid modernity. That the response of HSWs tends to be at the individual level is not surprising, since individualisation is a hallmark of liquid modern society.

The approach of the HSWs in this study is, to a certain extent, well adapted to some of the challenges of old age in liquid modernity. Where the physical and mental illnesses of old age begin to diminish the abilities of older people to engage in life politics, social workers are in a position to protect the availability of choices and the power of individuals to make them. This is a key aspect of the HSWs' practices. Of crucial importance is the fact that the HSWs' defining principle of self-determination is accompanied by a willingness to provide a muscular form of advocacy that can have a tangible impact in achieving the outcome desired by the patient or carers. In focusing their efforts to achieve objectives defined by the patient, HSWs therefore practice in an emancipatory fashion. Of course, there are limits to the power of HSWs as an emancipatory force. The HSWs' conception of human rights as primarily negative rights means that there are those to whom their help will not extend, since the HSWs are not in a position to engage with the social and structural factors that prevent some patients from taking advantage of their full rights. Engagement in life politics is not possible for those whose lives are blighted by oppression and inequality (Garrett, 2004), meaning that the promotion of choices may be meaningless to some older people.

The willingness of HSWs to advocate for positive risk-taking on behalf of patients is a significant demonstration of the potential of social workers to assist older people through the challenges of 'liquid' old age. Physical frailty, progressive dementia and the risk of falls are all aspects of patients' post-discharge lives that bring great uncertainty not only to the individual affected, but to her/his family. HSWs often therefore encounter relatives or carers who wish to see their loved one in the safety of residential care or receiving the maximum possible number of house calls from community care services. Where this is in opposition to what the patient wants, the advocacy of HSWs not only promotes the patient's choice but may also help family members to come to terms with the uncertainties that will arise from respecting the patient's choices. In so doing, HSWs often have a role to play in challenging ageist assumptions about the quality of life older people can expect to have, and their right to self-determination (Ray and Phillips, 2012).

Just as the HSWs work in a way that assists older people to face some of the 'liquid' challenges that old age produces, they also assist older people and their families to cope with balancing the need of the patient for long-term care with the need of working-age people to be flexible and responsive to the demands of the labour market. HSWs create their care plans through establishing the wishes of the patient (or what is considered to be in their best interests if they lack mental capacity), what any informal carers are able to do, and what services the patient might be eligible to receive. This means that care planning can be responsive to the situation of the patient and her/his family circumstances. Care planning is therefore an activity that is useful to the neoliberal economy, yet it should not be condemned as a social work practice, as some suggest (e.g. Hastings and Rogowski, 2015; Penna and O'Brien, 2013; Garrett, 2004), because of its complicity in the form of capitalism that is widely held responsible for the inequalities and disadvantages that social work strives to correct. Whatever economic policies a state might pursue, as long as it assumes responsibility for the welfare of its citizens, some form of care planning for individual older people will always be required. Acknowledgement of this points again to the necessity of refining social work's understanding of itself so that social work roles that focus only on the micro level are not regarded as falling short of the ideal.

It must be acknowledged that, when social workers advocate positive risk-taking and stand up for the rights of individual patients to make choices about their discharge destinations and care plans, they are not only articulating and enacting the values of liquid modernity and responding to needs created by the lifestyles of liquid modernity, but also facilitating the reproduction of 'liquid old age', since the result of taking positive risks is often further uncertainty. As was noted in Chapter 6, the care plans made by social workers for extremely frail older people to return to their homes may only postpone an inevitable need for residential care by a few weeks or months. Many such care plans come to an end when an older person has a further hospital admission due to a fall or some other unmanageable decline in their health. There is a fine distinction to be drawn between practices that are liberating in promoting individual choice, and those which abandon people to their fate, by leaving them with full responsibility for dealing with the circumstances beyond their control.

In arguing that the work of the HSWs represents a response to issues arising from liquid modernity, I reject the notion that social work is entirely in thrall to neoliberal ideology. In the processes of making assessments and creating care plans, the HSWs do engage in bureaucratic practices that are shaped by the neoliberal policy of community care, with its purchaser–provider split, emphasis on best value and managerial control. In the context of promoting personal choice and enabling individuals' engagement in life politics, however, community care might be seen not as a 'straitjacket' (Lymbery, 2010), but as an imperfect tool through which the aims of social work are delivered. The bureaucratic structures of community care may be dehumanising at times, and the HSWs admittedly do carry out some practices that have been identified as dehumanising, yet the bureaucratic system is not capable of dehumanising the HSWs' work entirely. The highly rationalised nature of the bureaucratic system is kept in check by the HSWs' empathy for patients and carers and by their clear sense that their loyalty remains with the individual patient, rather than with the bureaucracy.

The HSWs' values share roots with neoliberalism in terms of the liberal tradition of respect for negative freedoms (Banks, 2012) yet, while the accomplishment of prompt patient discharges may serve the purpose demanded by neoliberal governments, the HSWs tend to be motivated primarily by regard for the welfare of the individual patient, rather than efficiency and saving the state money. The HSWs' assertion of their independence within the hospital setting, explored in Chapter 7, is suggestive of an occupational group with a clear sense of values and a clear purpose. HSWs' self-claimed role as advocates for patients might even be interpreted as an assertion of liquid modern values – those of self-determination and personal responsibility for one's own fate – within a setting that is still grounded in solid modernity, with its certainties of professional hierarchies, the dominance of medical knowledge and the expected relationship between patient and clinician. The HSWs assert their independence from clinicians for a purpose that is intrinsic to themselves and is derived from their professional and personal values, distinguishing them markedly from adherents of bureaucracies along the lines of the classic Weberian model,

> in which identities and social bonds were deposited on entry in the cloakroom together with hats, umbrellas and overcoats, so that solely the command and the statute book could drive, uncontested, the actions of the insiders as long as they stayed inside.
>
> (Bauman, 2000a, pp. 25–26)

Although a large part of their work involves the operation of a bureaucratic system, and despite a managerial system that is partially able to control their everyday work, HSWs work to an identifiable set of values that is beyond the control of bureaucratic or managerial systems. As street-level bureaucrats (Lipsky, 1980), they retain discretion in the way they carry out their work, yet they use this discretion not only to control their workload in ways that protect their own interests, as Lipsky suggested, but also at times to engage in the deeper complexities with which they are confronted in the lives of patients. While the bureaucratic nature of their work influences their interactions with patients, the solutions for problems they can offer and even the nature of issues with which they concern themselves, by orientating their practices around their professional and personal values, HSWs retain the power over defining their own aims.

When defining their aims, the HSWs almost always regard promoting the welfare of the individual patient as their primary concern. In this, there appears to be some dissonance with the way social work as a profession has attempted to define its own nature. The IFSW's definition of social work, with its emphasis on social change and engagement with structures, and the continued currency of ideas derived from radical social work throughout social work scholarship, suggest that working only at the level of the individual is not enough. This is unfair to social workers in roles such as that of the HSWs involved in this study. The nature of the tasks they are employed to complete is unsuited to extensive engagement with the wider social forces that shape the lives of patients and carers. Further, social workers in the UK are working in a country that has chosen through the ballot box governments that favour neoliberalism since 1979. While social workers and social work academics may have valid and profound concerns about the policies adopted by their governments, it is not realistic to expect social workers to effect political and social change against the tide of popular political discourse. As was noted in Chapter 2, social work can trace its origins to two separate strands: the casework approach introduced by the Charity Organisation Society and the more collectivist approach of the Settlement movement. The tension between these two sides of social work has never been fully resolved and is perpetuated through ongoing debates between the more individually orientated theory of anti-discriminatory practice and the more structurally focused anti-oppressive practice (Thompson, 2016; Dominelli, 2002). A more nuanced definition of social work is therefore needed, that recognises that both the individually focused, liberal practice typified by the HSWs, and radical practices that overtly aim towards wider social and structural change, have their place.

The values and practices of the HSWs are largely in harmony with the zeitgeist of liquid modernity, with its emphasis on personal choice and responsibility for one's own fate. The values of the HSWs are characterised by a liberalism that hinges on respect for the individual and her/his right to self-determination. While managerial and bureaucratic control shape the everyday practices of the HSWs and impose some limits on the extent to which they can engage with patients and their families, ultimately the HSWs' practices are driven by their values. The strength of the HSWs' identity within the hospital and the coherence of their own distinct frame of understanding is indicative of an occupational group that has a clear sense of its own purpose and confidence in the values underpinning its practices. The lack of regular engagement beyond the micro level seen in social work teams in this sort of role should not be regarded as a failure – instead, the realities of social work practice in neoliberal states should be allowed for in a more nuanced understanding of the nature of social work than the IFSW's definition suggests.

Future directions

Discharge planning

There is no legal obligation for local authorities to base teams in hospitals, and not all do. If nothing else, the empirical research that I have undertaken confirms the importance of having social workers based in hospitals for the purposes of discharge planning. Although hospital social work and community-based care management have much in common, and hospital social work could not be said to be a specialism in terms of expert knowledge or qualification, hospital social work does require a specialised skillset in terms of making rapid assessments, managing sometimes fraught relations with and between patients, carers and health professionals, and managing a high caseload with a fast turnover. Demand for discharge planning services is likely to rise with the growth of the ageing population noted in Chapter 1 and it is vital that social work continues to be able to offer rapid and flexible responses to hospital patients' social care needs. It is particularly important that qualified social workers, who have developed a due regard for human rights, social justice and empowerment, are at the centre of discharge planning to advocate for patients' and families' choices. It would be all too easy for discharge processes to become dominated by the needs of service providers, which in turn would be likely to give rise to more instrumental, dehumanising approaches to moving patients on from hospital care.

As noted above, the practice of hospital social work described in my research seems somewhat removed from the IFSW's ambitious, if rather abstract, definition of social work. Davies (1985; 1994) argued that, far from being a force for creating profound social change, social work's purpose is to maintain stability in an unequal society through providing assistance to its most vulnerable members, and held hospital social work up as a prime example of the maintenance role. Clearly, it is the everyday business of HSWs to help individuals to adjust to circumstances caused by and/or impacting on their health, rather than to engage in attempts to challenge wider structures and power relations. Doing so, however, frequently involves HSWs assisting patients or carers to challenge the people or systems that have power over them. Rather than being 'maintenance mechanics oiling the interpersonal wheels of the community' (Davies, 1985, p. 31), then, we might see social workers engaged in discharge planning work as mechanics who are continually adjusting and reconfiguring select elements of the machinery of society. This might not lead to profound structural changes, but it does mean that HSWs have at least some limited ability to influence the overall direction of travel. That is to say, even when social work is focused only on helping an individual adjust to her/his circumstances, social workers are obliged to take a stance of either accepting or challenging the social forces that act upon that individual. In Mills' ([1959] 2000) terms, through assisting people with personal troubles, HSWs make an impact on public issues.

Hospital social work, then, is not an activity that can be neutral towards social forces and structures and therefore practitioners ought to cultivate insight into the ways in which their actions either maintain and reproduce power relations or alter them, however subtly. As I outlined in Chapter 4, critical engagement with such issues requires that HSWs draw upon both research and theory and do not rely on practice experience alone. Ferguson's (2008) model of critical best practice is helpful in this regard because it allows for social workers to draw on a wide and varied range of empirical and theoretical perspectives in interpreting their own practice experiences. For example, discharge planning should be founded upon the principle that individuals and families have the right to choose how to live their own lives, yet the hospital social work role cannot be regarded as a simple matter of advocacy and wish fulfilment. From a theoretical perspective, critical gerontology can help HSWs to understand the ways through which a lifetime of marginalisation, disadvantage and oppression may influence individuals towards irrational or self-destructive choices (Ray et al., 2015). Alongside this theoretical understanding, emerging research evidence suggests that, though there is a strong tendency for older people who require care to choose to remain in their own homes rather than move to residential or even 'extra care' provisions, people who receive domiciliary care in their own homes feel less in control and less satisfied than those in 'extra care' or residential care (Callaghan and Towers, 2014; Phillips et al., 2015; Boyle, 2004). It is not for HSWs to draw on this theoretical and empirical knowledge to claim that they know best for people in the planning process, but rather to use these forms of knowledge to guide relational work in which the context of individual and family life stories is acknowledged and people are fully supported at moments of life transition (Phillips and Waterson, 2005). Discharge planning may result in older people and their carers living with increasing uncertainty and risk, or in making a significant and permanent change in lifestyle, and they therefore need HSWs to engage them in thinking through the potential consequences of their choices and planning for contingencies.

For HSWs, the insights of critical gerontology are particularly important for challenging the age-based discrimination so often experienced by older hospital patients and for subverting the view that frailty or dependency are indications of personal failure (Lloyd, 2014). Common understandings of old age as characterised by deficits and impairment, which act as markers of unbecoming and reduced personhood (Gilleard and Higgs, 2010) must be challenged. This means that all older people's social workers need to develop perspectives that recognise the value of people notwithstanding their ability to exercise individual action or intentionality (Grenier et al., 2017). Social work education is not yet doing enough to encourage qualifying social workers to engage with critical theories of ageing (Richards et al., 2014), yet the increase in the ageing population brings an urgent need for social workers to develop their understanding of ageing within contemporary society.

Health-related social work

While discharge planning will remain an important social work activity, the growth of the ageing population in the coming years means that health and social care services will need to transform themselves. The rising costs of critical and acute health care for older people would suggest that there is an urgent need for interventions that will help people to avoid requiring hospital care as much as possible. Meeting this objective will involve an approach to social work with older people that encompasses not merely responding to the presentation of unmet care needs, but actively engaging with older people to help them to find ways to cope with the difficulties of chronic illnesses and mental and physical decline before their situation becomes critical. There is potential for hospital social work to move beyond being confined to a reactive service for those in crisis and to play a fuller role in enhancing people's health and well-being. This implies expanding the scope of health-related social work within both hospital and community-based teams.

The knowledge and skills of contemporary social workers in the UK are well suited to an expanded role in engaging with people to promote lifestyle and behavioural changes to enhance health and well-being. Systems theory, strengths-based approaches, solution-focused therapy, motivational interviewing and task-centred work can all be readily adapted to assist people to cope with and manage health conditions. Additionally, the developing model of health coaching (Palmer et al., 2003; Lindner et al., 2003; Olsen, 2014) may provide a fruitful applied theoretical framework for direct work with people to manage health needs. At the heart of health coaching is the suggestion that practitioners assist people to mobilise their internal strengths and access external resources in order to achieve self-determined goals (Olsen, 2014). Such an approach is very much in harmony with the social work values of empowerment, social justice and human rights and could feasibly be incorporated by social workers in developing work with people with chronic health conditions and others whose health is vulnerable whether due to ageing or previous lifestyle choices.

As noted in Chapter 3, several studies in the USA and Australia in recent years (e.g. Alvarez, et al., 2016; Barber et al., 2015; Bronstein et al., 2015; Simpson et al., 2016; Cleak and Turczynski, 2014) have successfully explored the potential of HSWs to reduce rates of readmission to hospital. In undertaking this work, HSWs have retained their involvement in planning the care patients will receive after discharge, but have added therapeutic and educational interventions that aim to help patients to adapt psychologically to their circumstances and to develop behaviours that may protect them from further deteriorations of their health, whether caused by disease progression or accident. An important underlying assumption in these schemes is that a hospital admission is often not a single, isolated health incident, but rather the result of a combination of physical, social, psychological and emotional states, and that a hospital discharge should be regarded as a staged process rather than a single moment of change. This holistic approach to understanding older people's health and the management of risk of future admissions draws more fully on the knowledge base of social work than the narrower approach to discharge planning common in the UK. It requires practitioners who are skilled in interpersonal work and knowledgeable in implementing therapeutic interactions. The evidence from the fieldwork I report on in this book is that UK HSWs do retain an impressive range of interactional skills that could be mobilised for therapeutic purposes given the opportunity.

If the UK is to emulate the successes of the American and Australian hospital social work schemes, it will be necessary to provide evidence that they offer added value for money. There will be pitfalls in assessing the financial viability of enhanced social work interventions. Since the NHS and local authorities hold budgets independently of each other, co-operative partnership arrangements between management systems will be essential. Both the NHS and local authority social care services have been severely impaired by almost a decade of austerity measures, meaning that it will be difficult to persuade budget holders on both sides that this area is most worth prioritising. At managerial level, there is a need for recognition that high rates of readmission for older people represent a fixable area of wasted spending. Currently, NHS and local authority management systems do not track readmission rates for older people as a key performance indicator, yet this is the most obvious measure of how enhanced hospital social work interventions might provide cost savings to the NHS. Of greater significance is that a reduction in hospital readmissions might also be understood to correlate with a reduction in human suffering. A word of caution must be added, however. Prioritising a reduction of rates of readmission to hospital must not be allowed to drive a more risk-averse approach to care planning by social workers that would reduce patients' freedom of choice about the life they will live after discharge.

Providing evidence that enhanced social work interventions within hospitals offer added value for money will require the production of some research outputs that could be seen to answer the question 'What works?'. As noted in Chapter 4, a simplistic approach to 'What works?' is not satisfactory for social work, yet evidence regarding the efficacy of social work interventions can contribute fulsomely to critical best practice. Hospital social work will need to take a pragmatic approach to investigating the outcomes of enhanced interventions with older people – one that can produce the kinds of messages that policy-makers and senior managers need in order to justify committing their funds, while at the same time ensuring that social work's wider priorities are not overlooked. In other words, appraisal of HSWs' interventions should measure instrumental aims such as reduction in readmission rates (and the consequent saving to the NHS) while also ensuring that the lived experiences of patients and carers are improved. This means that HSWs need to be involved in the design and conduct of the research, developing the role of the practitioner-researcher. Involving HSWs as practitioner-researchers in schemes of action research will ensure that HSWs are able to drive the developments that they want to see and may also enhance their professional standing among their clinician colleagues. This, in turn, will strengthen the position of social workers as advocates for patients.

Hospital social workers play a valuable role in planning the care of people with complex social and health needs, balancing the necessity to accomplish discharges as quickly as possible with an insistence on protecting the best interests and choices of individuals. Even in the highly bureaucratised context of the UK, HSWs maintain a distinct professional identity and find ways to enact the values of human rights, social justice and empowerment. More use could be made of their knowledge and skills to reduce rates of readmission to hospital through the delivery of programmes to help people to learn to manage their health. As more people live into advanced old age, higher numbers will be living with chronic health conditions and in need of social care. It is vital that social workers contribute a perspective that is informed by critical gerontology and research both to hospital discharge planning and to developing interventions that promote health-protective behaviours in older people.

References

Abbott, A. (1988). *The System of Professions: An Essay on the Division of Expert Labour*. Chicago, IL: University of Chicago Press.

Abramson, J.S. and Mizrahi, T. (1996). 'When Social Workers and Physicians Collaborate: Positive and Negative Interdisciplinary Experiences', *Social Work*, 41(3), pp. 270–281.

Adams, R. (2008). *Empowerment, Participation and Social Work*. 4th Edition. Basingstoke, UK: Palgrave Macmillan.

Age UK (2011). *Older People and Human Rights: A Reference Guide for Professionals Working with Older People*. London: Age UK/BIHR.

Age UK (2017). *Briefing: Health and Care of Older People in England 2017*. Available at: http://www.ageuk.org.uk/Documents/EN-GB/For-professionals/Research/The_Health_and_Care_of_Older_People_in_England_2016.pdf?dtrk=true [Accessed 9/2/20].

Albrithen, A. and Yalli, N. (2015). 'Hospital Social Workers in Saudi Arabia: Characteristics and Functions', *Social Work in Health Care*, 54(2), pp. 158–176.

Albrithen, A. and Yalli, N. (2016). 'Social Workers: Peer Interaction and Hospital Integration', *International Social Work*, 59(1), pp. 129–140.

Allen, D. (1997). 'The Nursing-medical Boundary: A Negotiated Order?', *Sociology of Health and Illness*, 19(4), pp. 498–520.

Allen, R. (2014). *The Role of the Social Worker in Adult Mental Health Services*. London, UK: College of Social Work.

Alvarez, R., Ginsburg, J., Grabowski, J., Post, S. and Rosenberg, W. (2016). 'The Social Work Role in Reducing 30 Day Readmissions: The Effectiveness of the Bridge Model of Transitional Care', *Journal of Gerontological Social Work*, 59(3), pp. 222–227.

Atkinson, P. A. (1995). *Medical Talk and Medical Work: The Liturgy of the Clinic*. London: Sage.

Auerbach, C., Mason, S. E. and Laporte, H. H. (2007). 'Evidence that Supports the Value of Social Work in Hospitals', *Social Work in Health Care*, 44(1), pp. 17–32.

Baars, J. (1991). 'The Challenge of Critical Gerontology: The Problem of Social Constitution', *Journal of Ageing Studies*, 5(3), pp. 219–243.

Baltes, P. (1997). 'On the Incomplete Architecture of Human Ontogeny: Selection, Optimization and Compensation as a Foundation of Developmental Theory', *American Psychologist*, 52(4), pp. 366–380.

Banks, S. (2012). *Ethics and Values in Social Work*. 4th Edition. Basingstoke, UK: Palgrave Macmillan.

Barber, R.D., Coulourides Kogan, A., Riffenburgh, A. and Enguidanos, S. (2015). 'A Role for Social Workers in Improving Care Setting Transitions: A Case Study', *Social Work in Health Care*, 54(3), pp. 177–192.

Barnett, S.A. and Barnett, D.H.O.W. (1915). *Practicable Socialism*. London, UK: Longmans, Green & Co.

Barry, A.M. and Yuill, C. (2016). *Understanding the Sociology of Health*. 4th Edition. London, UK: Sage.

Bass, C. and Halligan, P. (2014). 'Factitious Disorders and Malingering: Challenges for Clinical Assessment and Management', *The Lancet*, 383(9926), pp. 1422–1432. doi:10.1016/S0140–6736(13)62186–62188

Basso Lipani, M., Holster, K. and Bussey, S. (2015). 'The Preventable Admissions Care Team (PACT): A Social Work-Led Model of Transitional Care', *Social Work in Health Care*, 54(9), pp. 810–827.

Bauman, Z. (1989). *Modernity and the Holocaust*. Cambridge, UK: Polity.

Bauman, Z. (2000a). *Liquid Modernity*. Cambridge, UK: Polity.

Bauman, Z. (2000b). 'Special Essay – Am I my Brother's Keeper?', *European Journal of Social Work*, 3(1), pp. 5–11.

Bauman, Z. (2007). *Liquid Times: Living in an Age of Uncertainty*. Cambridge, UK: Polity.

Beck, U., Giddens, A. and Lash, S. (1994). *Reflexive Modernisation: Politics, Traditions and Aesthetics in the Modern Social Order*. Cambridge, UK: Polity.

Becker, H.S. (1961). *Boys in White: Student Culture in Medical School*. Chicago, IL: Chicago University Press.

Beckett, C. and Maynard, A. (2013). *Values and Ethics in Social Work*. London, UK: Sage.

Beddoe, L. (2011). 'Health Social Work: Professional Identity and Knowledge', *Qualitative Social Work*, 12(1), pp. 24–40.

Bellamy, J., Bledsoe, S.E. and Traube, D. (2006). 'The Current State of Evidence Based Practice in Social Work: A Review of the Literature and Qualitative Analysis of Expert Interviews', *Journal of Evidence-Based Social Work*, 3, pp. 23–48.

Benson, R.T., Drew J.C. and Galland, R.B. (2006). 'A Waiting List to Go Home: An Analysis of Delayed Discharges from Surgical Beds', *Annals of the Royal College of Surgeons*, 88(7), pp. 650–652.

Berger, P. and Luckmann, T. (1967). *The Social Construction of Reality*. London, UK: Allen Lane.

Bernard, M., Phillipson, C. and Phillips, J. (2001). 'Continuity and Change in the Family and Community Life of Older People', *Journal of Applied Gerontology*, 20(3), pp. 259–278.

Bevan, A. (1952). *In Place of Fear*. London, UK: Heinemann.

Boutwell, A.E., Johnson, M.B. and Watkins, M.S. (2016). 'Analysis of a Social Work-Based Model of Transitional Care to Reduce Hospital Readmissions: Preliminary Data', *Journal of the American Geriatrics Society*, 64, pp. 1104–1107.

Boyle, G. (2004). 'Facilitating Choice and Control for Older People in Long-term Care', *Health and Social Care in the Community*, 12(3), pp. 212–220.

Bradby, H. (2009). *Medical Sociology: An Introduction*. London, UK: Sage.

Brake, M. and Bailey, R. (eds.) (1975). *Radical Social Work and Practice*. London, UK: Edward Arnold.

Brewer, C. and Lait, J. (1980). *Can Social Work Survive?* London, UK: Temple Smith.

Broadhurst, K., Wastell, D., White, S., Hall, C., Peckover, S., Thompson, K., Pithouse, A. and Davey, D. (2010). 'Performing "Initial Assessment": Identifying the Latent Conditions for Error at the Front-door of Local Authority Children's Services', *British Journal of Social Work*, 40(2), pp. 352–370.

Bronstein, L.R., Gould, P., Berkowitz, S.A., James, G.D. and Marks, K. (2015). 'Impact of a Social Work Care Coordination Intervention on Hospital Readmission: A Randomized Controlled Trial', *Social Work*, 60(3), pp. 248–255.

Burnett, P. J. (1994). *Idle Hands: The Experience of Unemployment, 1790–1990*. London, UK: Routledge.

Burns, T. (1992). *Irving Goffman*. London, UK: Routledge.

Butler, J. (2009). *Frames of War: When is Life Grievable?* London, UK: Verso.

Butrym, Z. (1967). *Social Work and Medical Care*. London, UK: Routledge and Kegan Paul.

Bywaters, P., McLeod, E. and Cooke, M. (2002). 'A Diversionary Tactic? Social Work in an Emergency Assessment Unit', *Nursing Older People*, 14(1), pp. 19–21.

Callaghan, L. and Towers, A.M. (2014). 'Feeling in Control: Comparing Older People's Experiences in Different Care Settings', *Ageing and Society*, 34(8), pp. 1427–1451.

Calnan, M., Tadd, W., Calnan, S., Hillman, A., Read, S. and Bayer, A. (2013). '"I Often Worry About the Older Person Being in That System": Exploring the Key Influences on the Provision of Dignified Care for Older People in Acute Hospitals', *Ageing and Society*, 33(3), pp. 465–485.

Campbell, J. and Oliver, M. (1996). *Disability Politics: Understanding our past, changing our future*. Abingdon, UK: Routledge.

Cannon, I. M. (1913). *Social Work in Hospitals: A Contribution to Progressive Medicine*. London, UK: Russell Sage Foundation.

Carey, M. (2015). 'The Fragmentation of Social Work and Social Care: Some Ramifications and a Critique', *British Journal of Social Work*, 45(8), pp. 2406–2422.

Carr, S. and Robbins, D. (2009). *The Implementation of Individual Budget Schemes in Adult Social Care: Research Briefing 20*. London, UK: Social Care Institute for Excellence.

Challis, D., Hughes, J., Chengqiu, X. and Jolley, D. (2014). 'An Examination of Factors Influencing Delayed Dscharge of Older People from Hospital', *International Journal of Geriatric Psychiatry*, 29, pp. 160–168.

Chalmers, I. (2003), 'Trying to Do More Good than Harm in Policy and Practice: The Role of Rigorous, Transparent, Up-to-date Evaluations', *Annals of the American Academy of Political and Social Science*, 589, pp. 22–40.

Chan, W.C.H. (2014). 'Relationships between Psycho-social Issues and Physical Symptoms of Hong Kong Chinese Palliative Care Patients: Insights into Social Workers' Role in Symptoms Management', *British Journal of Social Work*, 44(8), pp. 2342–2359.

Charmaz, K. (2014). *Constructing Grounded Theory*. 2nd Edition. London, UK: Sage.

Charmaz, K. and Brynant, A. (2016). 'Constructing Grounded Theory Analyses', in D. Silverman (ed.), *Qualitative Research*. 4th Edition. London, UK: Sage.

Clark, C.L. (2000). *Social Work Ethics*. Basingstoke, UK: Palgrave Macmillan.

Clarke, J. and Newman, J. (1997). *The Managerial State*. London: Sage.

Cleak, H.M. and Turczynski, M. (2014). 'Hospital Social Work in Australia: Emerging Trends or More of the Same?', *Social Work in Health Care*, 53(3), pp. 199–213.

Cloke, P., Goodwin, M. and Milbourne, P. (1997). *Rural Wales: Community and Marginalization*. Cardiff, UK: University of Wales Press.

Collins, R. (2004). *Interaction Ritual Chains*. Princeton, NJ: Princeton University Press.

Connor, A. and Tibbitt, J. (1988). *Social Workers and Health Care in Hospitals*. Edinburgh, UK: HMSO.

Coulshed, V., Mullender, A., Jones, D.N. and Thompson, N. (2006). *Management in Social Work*. 3rd Edition. Basingstoke, UK: Palgrave.

Craig, S. L. and Muskat, B. (2013). 'Bouncers, Brokers and Glue: The Self-described Roles of Social Workers in Urban Hospitals', *Health and Social Work*, 38(1), pp. 7–17.

Craig, S.L., Betancourt, I. and Muskat, B. (2015). 'Thinking Big, Supporting Families and Enabling Coping: The Values of Social Work in Patient and Family Centred Health Care', *Social Work in Health Care*, 54(5), pp. 422–443.

Cullen, L.T. (2013). 'The First Lady Almoner: The Appointment, Position, and Findings of Miss Mary Stewart at the Royal Free Hospital, 1895–1899', *Journal of the History of Medicine and Allied Sciences*, 68(4), pp. 551–582.

Dahlberg, L., Demack, S. and Bambra, C. (2007). 'Age and Gender of Informal Carers: A Population-based Study in the UK', *Health and Social Care in the Community*, 15(5), pp. 439–445.

Davies, M. (1985). *The Essential Social Worker: A Guide to Positive Practice*. 2nd Edition. Aldershot, UK: Gower Publishing Company.

Davies, M. (1994). *The Essential Social Worker: An Introduction to Professional Practice in the 1990s*. 3rd Edition. Farnham, UK: Ashgate.

Davis, C. (2004). 'Hospital Social Work: Are We Conducting the Right Type of Research?' *Social Work in Health Care*, 38(1), pp. 67–79.

Davis, C., Milosevic, B., Baldry, E. and Walsh, A. (2004). 'Defining the Role of the Hospital Social Worker in Australia: Part 2 – A Qualitative Approach', *International Social Work*, 48(3), pp. 289–299.

De Montigny, G. (1995). *Social Working: An Ethnography of Frontline Practice*. Toronto, Canada: University of Toronto Press.

Dedman, G. (1996). '1946–1973: Reconstruction and Integration: Social Work in the National Health Service', in J. Baraclough, G. Dedman, H. Osborn and P. Willmott (eds.), *100 Years of Health Related Social Work*. Birmingham, UK: BASW.

Deeming, C. (2009). '"Active Ageing" in Practice: A Case Study in East London, UK', *Policy & Politics*, 37(1), pp. 93–111.

Degnen, C. (2007). 'Minding the Gap: The Construction of Old Age and Oldness among Peers', *Journal of Aging Studies*, 21(1), pp. 69–80.

Delamont, S. and Atkinson, P. (1995). *Fighting Familiarity: Essays on Education and Ethnography*. Cresskill, NJ: Hampton Press.

Delamont, S., Atkinson, P. and Pugsley, L. (2010). 'The Concept Smacks of Magic: Fighting Familiarity Today', *Teaching and Teacher Education*, 26(1), pp. 3–10.

Denzin, N.K. and Lincoln, Y.S. (eds.) (2011). *The SAGE Handbook of Qualitative Research*. 4th Edition. London, UK: Sage.

Department for Constitutional Affairs (2007). *Mental Capacity Act 2005 Code of Practice*. London, UK: TSO.

Department of Health (1992). *Social Services for Hospital Patients. Part 1: Working at the Interface*. London, UK: HMSO.

Department of Health (2008). *Personalisation*. Archived at: http://webarchive.nationala rchives.gov.uk/+/www.dh.gov.uk/en/SocialCare/Socialcarereform/Personalisation/DH_ 080573 [Accessed 9/2/20].

Dewing, J. and Dijk, S. (2016). 'What is the Current State of Care for Older People with Dementia in General Hospitals? A Literature Review', *Dementia*, 15(1), pp. 106–124.

Dingwall, R. (1977). *The Social Organisation of Health Visitor Training*. London, UK: Croom Helm.

Doel, M. (2012). *Social Work: The Basics*. Abingdon, UK: Routledge.

Dominelli, L. (1996). 'Deprofessionalizing Social Work: Anti-Oppressive Practice, Competencies and Postmodernism', *British Journal of Social Work*, 26(2), pp. 153–175.

Dominelli, L. (2002). *Anti-oppressive Social Work Theory and Practice*. Basingstoke, UK: Palgrave Macmillan.

Dominelli, L. (2004). *Social Work: Theory and Practice for a Changing Profession*. Cambridge: Polity.

Dominelli, L. and Hoogvelt, A. (1996). 'Globalization and the Technocratization of Social Work', *Critical Social Policy*, 47(1), pp. 45–62.

Donnellon, A., Gray, B. and Bougon, M. (1986). 'Communication, Meaning and Organized Action', *Administrative Science Quarterly*, 31(1), pp. 43–55.

Drakeford, M. (2005). 'Health Policy in Wales: Making a Difference in Conditions of Difficulty', *Critical Social Policy*, 26(3), pp. 497–503.

Du Toit, A. (2012). *Making sense of 'Evidence': Thinking the relationship(s). between research and policymaking - Presentation to The politics of poverty research - learning from the practice of policy dialogue*. Available at: http://www.plaas.org.za/sites/default/files/publications-pdf/Du%20Toit%20%20Making%20sense%20of%20%27Evidence%27%202012%2011%20presentation.pdf [Accessed 1/7/13].

Dustin, D. (2007). *The McDonaldization of Social Work*. Farnham, UK: Ashgate.

Eccles, A. and Taylor, R. (2018). *Personalisation: Back to the Future? Reflections on the 1968 Act*. Edinburgh, UK: Social Work Scotland.

Ellis, K., Davis, A. and Rummery, K. (1999). 'Needs Assessment, Street-level Bureaucracy and the New Community Care', *Social Policy and Administration*, 33(3), pp. 262–280.

Evans, T. and Harris, J. (2004). 'Street-level Bureaucracy, Social Work and the (Exaggerated) Death of Discretion', *British Journal of Social Work*, 34(6), pp. 871–895.

Ferguson, H. (2003a). 'In Defence (and Celebration) of Individualization and Life Politics for Social Work', *British Journal of Social Work*, 33(5), pp. 699–707.

Ferguson, H. (2003b). 'Outline of a Critical Best Practice Perspective on Social Work and Social Care', *British Journal of Social Work*, 33(8), pp. 1005–1024.

Ferguson, H. (2007). *Reclaiming Social Work: Challenging Neo-liberalism and Promoting Social Justice*. London, UK: Sage.

Ferguson, H. (2008). 'The Theory and Practice of Critical Best Practice in Social Work', in K. Jones, B. Cooper and H. Ferguson (eds.), *Best Practice in Social Work: Critical Perspectives*. Basingstoke, UK: Palgrave Macmillan.

Ferguson, H. (2016). 'Researching Social Work Practice Close Up: Using Ethnographic and Mobile Methods to Understand Encounters between Social Workers, Children and Families', *British Journal of Social Work*, 46(1), pp. 153–168.

Ferlie, E., Ashburner, L., Fitzgerald, L. and Pettigrew, A. (1996). *The New Public Management in Action*. Oxford: Oxford University Press.

Fish, D. and Coles, C. (2000). 'Seeing Anew: Understanding Professional Practice as Artistry', *Changing Practice in Health and Social Care*. London: Sage.

Floersch, J., Longhofer, J. and Suskewicz, J. (2014). 'The Use of Ethnography in Social Work Research', *Qualitative Social Work*, 13(1), pp. 3–7.

Foucault, M. ([1975]1991). *Discipline and Punish: The Birth of the Prison*. Trans. A. Sheridan. London, UK: Penguin.

Foucault, M. (1982). 'Afterword: The Subject and Power', in H. Dreyfus and P. Rabinow (eds.), *Michel Foucault: Beyond Structuralism and Hermeneutics*. Chicago, IL: University of Chicago Press.

Foucault, M. (1984). 'On the Genealogy of Ethics: An Overview of Work in Progress', in P. Rabinow (ed.), *The Foucault Reader*. Harmondsworth, UK: Penguin.

Friedson, E. (1970). *The Profession of Medicine*. New York: Dodd Mead and Co.

Gambrill, E. (2001). 'Social Work: An Authority-based Profession', *Research on Social Work Practice*, 11(2), pp. 166–175.

Gardner, A. (2011). *Personalisation in Social Work*. Exeter, UK: Learning Matters.

Garrett, P.M. (2004). 'More Trouble with Harry: A Rejoinder in the "Life Politics" Debate', *British Journal of Social Work*, 34(4), pp. 577–589.

Gearing, R. E., Saini, M. and McNeill, T. (2007). 'Experiences and Implications of Social Workers Practicing in a Pediatric Hospital Environment Affected by SARS', *Health and Social Work*, 32(1), pp. 17–27.

Geertz, C. (1973). *The Interpretation of Cultures: Selected Essays*. New York, NY: Basic Books.

Gerdes, K.E. and Segal, E.A. (2009). 'A Social Work Model of Empathy', *Advances in Social Work*, 10(2), pp. 114–127.

Geyer, R. (2012). 'Can Complexity Move UK Policy beyond "Evidence-based Policy Making" and the "Audit Culture"? Applying a "Complexity Cascade" to Education and Health Policy', *Political Studies*, 60(1), pp. 20–43.

Gibbons, J. and Plath, D. (2006). '"Everybody Puts a Lot Into It!" Single Session Contacts in Hospital Social Work', *Social Work in Health Care*, 42(1), pp. 17–34.

Gibbons, J. and Plath, D. (2012). 'Single Session Social Work in Hospitals', *Australian and New Zealand Journal of Family Therapy*, 33(1), pp. 39–53.

Giddens, A. (1992). *The Transformation of Intimacy: Sexuality, Love and Eroticism in Modern Societies*. Cambridge, UK: Polity.

Giddens, A. (1998). *The Third Way: The Renewal of Social Democracy*. Cambridge, UK: Polity.

Giddens, A. (1999). *Runaway World: How Globalization is Reshaping Our Lives*. London, UK: Profile.

Giddens, A. and Sutton, P.W. (2017). *Sociology*. 8th Edition. Cambridge: Polity.

Gill, D. and Ingman, S. (1994). *Eldercare, Distributive Justice and the Welfare State: Retrenchment or Expandsion*. Albany, NY: Suny Press.

Gilleard, C. and Higgs, P. (2010). 'Aging without Agency: Theorizing the Fourth Age', *Aging & Mental Health*, 14(2), pp. 121–128.

Gilleard, C. and Higgs, P. (2011a). 'Aging, Abjection and Embodiment in the Fourth Age' *Journal of Aging Studies*, 25(2), pp. 135–142.

Gilleard, C. and Higgs, P. (2011b). 'Frailty, Disability and Old Age: A Re-appraisal', *Health*, 15(5), pp. 475–490.

Gillen, P. and Graffin, S. (2010). 'Nursing Delegation in the United Kingdom', *Online Journal of Issues in Nursing*, 15(2), Manuscript 6.

Gitlin, T. (1980). *The Whole World Is Watching: Mass Media in the Making and Unmaking of the New Left*. Berkley, CA: University of California Press.

Glasby, J. (2003). *Hospital Discharge: Integrating Health and Social Care*. Oxford, UK: Radcliffe Medical Press.

Glasby, J. and Lester, H. (2004). 'Delayed Hospital Discharge and Mental Health: The Policy Implications of Recent Research', *Social Policy and Administration*, 38(7), pp. 744–757.

Glasby, J., Littlechild, R. and Pryce, K. (2004). 'Show Me the Way to Go Home: A Narrative Review of the Literature on Delayed Hospital Discharges and Older People', *British Journal of Social Work*, 34(8), pp. 1189–1197.

Glaser, B.G. and Strauss, A.L. (1967). *The Discovery of Grounded Theory: Strategies for Qualitative Research.* Chicago, IL: Aldine Publishing.

Glendinning, C., Challis, D., Fernandez, J-L., Jacobs, S., Jones, K., Knapp, M., Manthorpe, J., Moran, N., Netten, A., Stevens, M. and Wilberforce, M. (2008). *Evaluation of the Individual Budgets Pilot Programme: Final Report.* York, UK: University of York Social Policy Research Unit.

Goffman, I. (1959). *The Presentation of Self in Everyday Life.* New York: Anchor.

Goffman, I. (1961). *Encounters: Two Studies in the Sociology of Interaction.* Indianapolis, IN: Bobbs-Merrill.

Goffman, I. (1974). *Frame Analysis: An Essay on the Organization of Experience.* New York: Harper and Row.

Goffman, I. (1981). *Forms of Talk.* Philadelphia, PA: University of Philadelphia Press.

Gorman, H. and Postle, K. (2003). *Transforming Community Care: A Distorted Vision?* Birmingham, UK: Venture.

Gosden, P.H. (1961). *The Friendly Societies in England, 1815–1875.* Manchester, UK: Manchester University Press.

Gouldner, A.W. (1970). *The Coming Crisis of Western Sociology.* New York, NY: Basic.

Grandey, A.A. (2003). 'When "The Show Must Go On": Surface Acting and Deep Acting as Determinants of Emotional Exhaustion and Peer-Rated Service Delivery', *Academy of Management Journal*, 46(1), pp. 86–96.

Grant, D.M. and Toh, J.S. (2017). 'Medical Social Work Positions: BSW or MSW?', *Social Work in Health Care*, 56(4), pp. 215–226.

Gray, A.M. (2013). *Transforming Adult Social Care in Northern Ireland: Personalisation.* Northern Ireland Assembly Briefing Paper <www>http://www.niassembly.gov.uk/globa lassets/documents/raise/knowledge_exchange/briefing_papers/gray020513.pdf [Accessed 28/11/19].

Gray, B., Purdy, J.M. and Ansari, S. (2015). 'From Interactions to Institutions: Microprocesses of Framing and Mechanisms for the Structuring of Institutional Fields', *Academy of Management Review*, 40(1), pp. 115–143.

Gray, M., Joy, E., Plath, D. and Webb, S. (2013). 'Implementing Evidence-Based Practice: A Review of the Empirical Research Literature', *Research on Social Work Practice*, 23, pp. 157–166.

Greener, J. (2015). 'Embedded Neglect, Entrenched Abuse: Market Failure and Mistreatment in Elderly Care', in Z. Irving, M. Fenger and J. Hudson (eds.), *Social Policy Review 27: Analysis and Debate in Social Policy 2015.* Bristol, UK: Policy Press.

Greenhalgh, T., Howick, J. and Maskrey, N. (2014). 'Evidence Based Medicine: A Movement in Crisis?', *British Medical Journal*, 348, g3725.

Greenwood, N. and McKenzie, A. (2010). 'Informal Caring for Stroke Survivors: Meta-ethnographic Review of Qualitative Literature', *Maturitas*, 66(3), pp. 268–276.

Gregory, R. (2001). 'Transforming Governmental Culture: A Sceptical View of the New Public Management', in T. Christensen and P. Laegreid (eds.), *New Public Management: The Transformation of Ideas and Practice.* Aldershot, UK: Ashgate Publishing Ltd.

Grenier A. (2012). *Transitions and the Life Course.* Bristol, UK: Policy Press.

Grenier, A. (2007). 'Constructions of Frailty in the English Language, Care Practice and the Lived Experience', *Ageing and Society*, 27(3), pp. 425–445.

Grenier, A. and Phillipson, C. (2013). 'Rethinking Agency in Late Life: Structural and Interpretive Approaches', in J. Baars, J. Dohmen, A. Grenier and C. Phillipson (eds.), *Ageing, Meaning and Social Structure.* Bristol, UK: Policy Press.

Grenier, A., Phillipson, C., Rudman, D.L., Hatzifilalithis, S., Kobayashi, K. and Marier, P. (2017). 'Precarity in Late Life: Understanding New Forms of Risk and Insecurity', *Journal of Aging Studies*, 43(1), pp. 9–14.

Griffiths Report (1988). *Community Care: Agenda for Action*. London, UK: HMSO.

Guba, E.G. and Lincoln, Y.S. (1994). 'Competing Paradigms in Qualitative Research', in N.K. Denzin and Y.S. Lincoln (eds.), *Handbook of Qualitative Research*. Thousand Oaks, CA: Sage.

Gunn, V., Muntaner, C., Ng, E., Villeneuve, M., Gea-Sanchez, M. and Chung, H. (2019). 'The Influence of Welfare State Factors on Nursing Professionalization and Nursing Human Resources: A Time-series Cross-sectional Analysis, 2000–2015', *Journal of Advanced Nursing*, 75, pp. 2797–2810.

Hamilton, C., Ronda, L., Hwang, U., Abraham, G., Baumlin, K., Morano, B., Nassisi, D. and Richardson, L. (2015). 'The Evolving Role of Geriatric Emergency Department Social Work in the Era of Health Care Reform', *Social Work in Health Care*, 54(9), pp. 849–868.

Hammersley M. (2005). 'Is the Evidence-based Practice Movement Doing More Good than Harm? Reflections on Iain Chalmers' Case for Research-based Policy Making and Practice', *Evidence & Policy*, 1(1). pp. 85–100.

Hammersley, M. (1992). *What's Wrong with Ethnography?* London, UK: Routledge.

Harlow, E. (2003). 'New Managerialism, Social Service Departments and Social Work Practice Today', *Practice*, 15(2), pp. 29–44.

Harris, J. (2003). *The Social Work Business*. London, UK: Routledge.

Harslof, I., Nielsen, U.S. and Feiring, M. (2017). 'Danish and Norwegian Hospital Social Workers' Cross-institutional Work Amidst Inter-sectoral Restructuring of Health and Social Welfare', *European Journal of Social Work*, 20(4), pp. 584–595.

Harvey, D. (2005). *A Brief History of Neoliberalism*. Oxford, UK: Oxford University Press.

Hasler, F. (2006). 'Holding the Dream: Direct Payments and Independent Living', in J. Leece and J. Bornat (eds.), *Developments in Direct Payments*. Bristol, UK: Policy Press.

Hastings, S.J. and Rogowski, S. (2015). 'Critical Social Work with Older People in Neo-liberal Times: Challenges and Critical Possibilities', *Practice – Social Work in Action*, 27(1), pp. 21–33.

Heenan, D. and Birrell, D. (2018). 'Hospital-Based Social Work: Challenges at the Interface between Health and Social Care', *British Journal of Social Work*, 49(7), pp. 1741–1758.

Helm, D. (2016). 'Sense-making in a Social Work Office: An Ethnographic Study of Safeguarding Judgements', *Child and Family Social Work*, 21(1), pp. 26–35.

Hennink, M., Hutter, I. and Bailey, A. (2011). *Qualitative Research Methods*. London: Sage.

Heywood, A. (2004). *Political Theory: An Introduction*. 3rd Edition. Basingstoke, UK: Palgrave Macmillan.

Higgs, P. and Gilleard, C. (2014). 'Frailty, Abjection and the "Othering" of the Fourth Age', *Health Sociology Review*, 23(1), pp. 10–19.

Hill, R., Betts, L.R. and Gardner, S.E. (2015). 'Older Adults' Experiences and Perceptions of Digital Technology: (Dis)empowerment, Wellbeing, and Inclusion', *Computers in Human Behaviour*, 48, pp. 415–423.

Hillman, A. and Latimer, J. (2017). 'Cultural Representations of Dementia', *Public Library of Science Medicine*, 14(3), e1002274.

Hillman, A., Tadd, W., Calnan, S., Calnan, M., Bayer, A. and Read, S. (2013). 'Risk, Governance and the Experience of Care', *Sociology of Health and Illness*, 35(6), pp. 939–955.

Hirsch, C.H., Sommers, L., Olsen, A., Mullen, L. and Winograd, C.H. (1990). 'The Natural History of Functional Morbidity in Hospitalized Older Patients', *Journal of the American Geriatric Society*, 38(12), pp. 1296–1303.

Hochschild, A. R. (2012). *The Managed Heart: Commercialization of Human Feeling.* Updated Edition. Berkeley, CA: University of California Press.

Holland, S., Burgess, S., Grogan-Kaylor, A. and Delva, J. (2011). 'Understanding Neighbourhoods, Communities and Environments: New Approaches for Social Work Research', *British Journal of Social Work*, 41(4), pp. 689–707.

Horlick-Jones, T. (2004). 'Editorial: Experts in Risk?... Do They Exist?'. *Health Risk and Scoiety*, 6(2), 107–114.

Hugman, R. (1991). *Power in Caring Professions.* Basingstoke, UK: Macmillan.

Hugman, R. (2009). 'But Is It Social Work? Some Reflections on Mistaken Identities', *British Journal of Social Work*, 39(6), pp. 1138–1153.

Humphries R. (2011). *Social Care Funding and the NHS: An Impending Crisis?* London, UK: Kings Fund.

Ife, J. (2010). *Human Rights from Below: Achieving Rights through Community Development.* Cambridge: Cambridge University Press.

Ife, J. (2012). *Human Rights and Social Work: Towards Rights-based Practice.* 3rd Edition. Cambridge: Cambridge University Press.

Illich, I., Irving, K.T., McKnight, J., Caplan, J. and Shaiken, H. (1977). *Disabling Professions.* London: Marion Boyers.

International Federation of Social Workers (IFSW) (2014). *Global Definition of Social Work.* Available at: http://ifsw.org/get-involved/global-definition-of-social-work/ [Accessed 6/10/17].

Isaksson, J., Lilliehorn, S. and Salander, P. (2017). 'A Nationwide Study of Swedish Oncology Social Workers: Characteristics, Clinical Functions, and Perceived Barriers to Optimal Functioning', *Social Work in Health Care*, 56(7), pp. 600–614.

Jackson, A.C., Johnson, B., O'Toole, M. and Auslander, G. (2001). 'Discharge Planning for Complex Paediatric Cases', *Social Work in Health Care*, 34(1–2), pp. 161–175.

Jenkins, N. (2014). 'Dementia and the Inter-embodied Self', *Social Theory and Health*, 12(2), pp. 125–137.

Johansson, S., Rosengren, A., Young, K. and Jennings, E. (2017). 'Mortality and Morbidity Trends after the First Year in Survivors of Acute Myocardial Infarction: A Systematic Review', *BMC Cardiovascular Disorders*, 17(1), 7 February, p. 53.

Johnson, T. J. (1972). *Professions and Power.* Basingstoke, UK: Macmillan.

Jordan, B. (1990). *Social Work in an Unjust Society.* Hemel Hempstead, UK: Harvester Wheatsheaf.

Judd, R.G. and Sheffield, S. (2010). 'Hospital Social Work: Contemporary Roles and Professional Activities', *Social Work in Health Care*, 49(9), pp. 856–871.

Kemp, E.S. (1912). 'The Training and Work of a Hospital Almoner', *The Hospital*, 52 (1349), 18 May, pp. 184–185.

Kennedy Chapin, R., Chandran, D., Sergeant, J.F. and Koenig, T.L. (2014). 'Hospital to Community Transitions for Adults: Discharge Planners' and Community Service Providers' Perspectives', *Social Work in Health Care*, 53(4), pp. 311–329.

Kidd, A.J. (1999). *State, Society, and the Poor in Nineteenth Century England.* Basingstoke, UK: Macmillan.

King's Fund (2014). *Making Our Health and Care Systems Fit for an Ageing Population*. London, UK: King's Fund.

Kitchen, A. and Brook, J. (2005). 'Social Work at the Heart of the Medical Team', *Social Work in Health Care*, 40(1), pp. 1–18.

Kitwood, T. (1997). *Dementia Reconsidered: The Person Comes First*. Buckingham, UK: Open University Press.

Klein, R. and Maybin, J. (2012). *Thinking about Rationing*. Available at: https://www.kingsfund.org.uk/sites/files/kf/field/field_publication_file/Thinking-about-rationing-the-kings-fund-may-2012.pdf [Accessed 16/3/17].

Kossman, H.D., Lamb, J.M., O'Brien, M.W., Predmore, S.M. and Prescher, M.J. (2006). 'Measuring Productivity in Medical Social Work', *Social Work in Health Care*, 42, pp. 1–16.

Kowalski, C., Ferencz, J., Weis, I., Adolph, H. and Weseelmann, S. (2015). 'Social Service Counselling in Cancer Centers Certified by the German Cancer Society', *Social Work in Health Care*, 54(4), pp. 307–319.

Laing, R. (1971). *The Politics of the Family and Other Essays*. London, UK: Routledge.

Lakey, L. (2009). *Counting the Cost: Caring for People with Dementia on Hospital Wards*. London, UK: Alzheimer's Society.

Larson, M.S. (1977). *The Rise of Professionalism*. Berkeley, CA: University of California Press.

Laslett, P. (1989). *A Fresh Map of Life: The Emergence of the Third Age*. Cambridge, MA: Harvard University Press.

Latimer, J. (2000). *The Conduct of Care: Understanding Nursing Practice*. Oxford, UK: Blackwell Science.

Leadbetter, C. (2004). *Personalisation Through Participation: A New Script for Public Services*. London, UK: Demos.

Lecompte, M.D. and Schensul, J.J. (1999). *Analyzing and Interpreting Ethnographic Data*. Lanham, MD: Altamira.

Leigh, C. (2004). *Unrepentant Whore: The Collected Work of Scarlot Harlot*. San Francisco, CA: Last Gasp.

Lewin, S. and Reeves, S. (2011). 'Enacting "Team" and "Teamwork": Using Goffman's Theory of Impression Management to Illuminate Interprofessional Practice on Hospital Wards', *Social Science and Medicine*, 72(10), pp. 1595–1602.

Lindner, H., Menzies, D., Kelly, J., Taylor, S. and Shearer, M. (2003). 'Coaching for Behaviour Change in Chronic Disease: A Review of the Literature and the Implications for Coaching as a Self-management Intervention', *Australian Journal of Primary Health*, 9(3), pp. 177–185.

Lipsky, M. (1980). *Street-Level Bureaucracy: The Dilemmas of Individuals in Public Services*. New York, NY: Russell Sage Foundation.

Lishman, J., Yuill, C., Brannan, J. and Gibson, A. (2018). *Social Work: An Introduction*. 2nd Edition. London, UK: Sage.

Lloyd, L., Tanner, D., Milne, A., Ray, M., Richards, S., Sullivan, M.P., Beech, C. and Phillips, J. (2014). 'Look After Yourself: Active Ageing, Individual Responsibility and the Decline of Social Work with Older People in the UK', *European Journal of Social Work*, 17(3), pp. 322–335.

Longhofer, J. and Floersch, J. (2012). 'An Example of Social Work Practice Ethnography', in S. Becker, A. Bryman and H. Ferguson (eds.), *Understanding Research for Social Policy and Social Work*. Bristol, UK: Policy Press.

Lowe, R. (2004). *The Welfare State in Britain since 1945*. 3rd Edition. Basingstoke, UK: Palgrave Macmillan.

Loxley, A. (1996). 'Training with the Institute of Almoners: 1958', in J. Baraclough, G. Dedman, H. Osborn and P. Willmott (eds.), *100 Years of Health Related Social Work*. Birmingham, UK: BASW.

Lymbery, M. (2001). 'Social Work at the Crossroads', *British Journal of Social Work*, 31(3), pp. 369–384.

Lymbery, M. (2005). *Social Work with Older People*. London, UK: Thousand Oaks.

Lymbery, M. (2010). 'A New Vision for Adult Social Care? Continuities and Change in the Care of Older People', *Critical Social Policy*, 30(1), pp. 5–26.

Lymbery, M. and Postle, K. (2010). 'Social Work in the Context of Adult Social Care in England and the Resultant Implications for Social Work Education', *British Journal of Social Work*, 40(8), pp. 2502–2522.

Lymbery, M. and Postle, K. (2015). *Social Work and the Transformation of Adult Services: Perpetuating a Distorted Vision?* Bristol, UK: Policy Press.

Macdonald, K.M. (1995). *The Sociology of the Professions*. London: Sage.

MacIntyre, A.C. (1981). *After Virtue: A Study in Moral Theory*. London, UK: Duckworth.

Macmillan (2014). *Cancer's Unequal Burden: The Reality behind Improving Cancer Survival Rates*. Available at: http://www.macmillan.org.uk/documents/cancersune qualburden_2014.pdf [Accessed 6/10/17].

Manchée, D.M. (1944). *Social Service in a General Hospital*. London, UK: Bailière, Tindall and Cox.

Manchée, D.M. (1945). 'The Social Aspect of the Venereal Diseases: The Work of the Almoner', *British Journal of Venereal Diseases*, 21, p. 12.

Mann, L. (2016). 'Delayed Discharges within Community Hospitals: A Qualitative Study Investigating the Perspectives of Frontline Health and Social Care Professionals', *Journal of Integrated Care*, 24(5/6), pp. 260–270.

Mantell, A. (2011). 'Human Rights and Wrongs: The Human Rights Act 1998', in T. Scragg and A. Mantell (eds.), *Safeguarding Adults in Social Work*. Exeter, UK: Learning Matters.

Manthorpe, J. (2002). 'Settlements and Social Work Education: Absorption and Accommodation', *Social Work Education*, 21, pp. 409–419.

Manzano-Santaella, A. (2010). 'From Bed-blocking to Delayed Discharges: Precursors and Interpretations of a Contested Concept', *Health Services Management Research*, 23, pp. 121–127.

Marsh, P. and Fisher, M. (2005). *Developing the Evidence Base for Social Work and Social Care Practice*. Bristol, UK: Policy Press/SCIE.

Matthews, J. and Kimmis, J. (2001). 'Development of the English Settlement Movement', in R. Gilchrist and T. Jeffs (eds.), *Settlements, Social Change and Community Action: Good Neighbours*. London, UK: Jessica Kingsley.

McDermott, F., Henderson, A. and Quayle, C. (2017). 'Health Social Workers' Sources of Knowledge for Decision Making in Practice', *Social Work in Health Care*, 56(9), pp. 794–808.

McDonald, A. (2006). *Understanding Community Care: A Guide for Social Workers*. 2nd Edition. Basingstoke, UK: Palgrave Macmillan.

McLaughlin, J. (2016). 'Social Work in Acute Hospital Settings in Northern Ireland: The Views of Service Users, Carers and Multi-disciplinary Professionals', *Journal of Social Work*, 16(2), pp. 135–154.

McNamee, S. and Hosking, D.M. (2012). *Research and Social Change: A Relational Constructionist Approach*. Abingdon, UK: Routledge.

Millar, M. (2008). '"Anti-oppressiveness": Critical Comments on a Discourse and its Context', *Journal of Social Work*, 38(2), pp. 362–375.

Mills, C.W. ([1959]2000). *The Sociological Imagination*. Oxford, UK: Oxford University Press.

Ministry of Justice (2008). *Deprivation of Liberty Safeguards: Code of Practice to Supplement the Main Mental Capacity Act 2005 Code of Practice*. London, UK: TSO.

Moberly Bell, E. (1961). *The Story of Hospital Almoners: The Birth of a Profession*. London, UK: Faber and Faber.

Morago, P. (2006). 'Evidence-based Practice: From Medicine to Social Work', *European Journal of Social Work*, 9(4), pp. 461–477.

Morgan, S. (1996). *Helping Relationships in Mental Health*. London, UK: Chapman and Hall.

Moriarty, J., Baginsky, M. and Manthorpe, J. (2015). *Literature Review of Roles and Issues within the Social Work Profession in England*. London, UK: King's College Social Care Workforce Research Unit.

Moriarty, J., Steils, N. and Manthorpe, J. (2019). *Mapping Hospital Social Work*. London, UK: NIHR Health and Social Care Workforce Research Unit, The Policy Institute at King's, King's College London.

Mosson, R., Hasson, H., Wallin, L. and von Thiele Schwarz, U. (2017). 'Exploring the Role of Line Managers in Implementing Evidence-based Practice in Social Services and Older People Care', *British Journal of Social Work*, 47(2), pp. 542–560.

Munro, E. (2011). *The Munro Review of Child Protection: Final Report, a Child-centred System*. London, UK: TSO.

Musil, L., Kubalcikova, K., Hubikova, O. and Necasova, M. (2004). 'Do social workers avoid the dilemmas of work with clients?', *European Journal of Social Work*, 7(3), pp. 305–319.

National Association of Social Workers (2017). *Qualified Clinical Social Worker – Information Booklet with Application and Reference Evaluation Forms*. Washington, DC: NASW.

National Audit Office (2016). *Discharging Older Patients from Hospital*. London, UK: NAO.

Nelson, M. (2000). 'A View of Social Work Advocacy in Hospitals in Eastern Ontario', *Social Work in Health Care*, 29, pp. 69–92.

Newman, T., Mosely, A., Tierney, S. and Ellis, A. (2005). *Evidence-based Social Work: A Guide for the Perplexed*. London, UK: Russell House.

NHS (2018a). *Decision Support Tool for NHS Continuing Healthcare*. Available at: https://www.gov.uk/government/publications/nhs-continuing-healthcare-decision-support-tool [Accessed 8/12/19].

NHS (2018b). *NHS Continuing Healthcare*. Available at: https://www.nhs.uk/conditions/social-care-and-support-guide/money-work-and-benefits/nhs-continuing-healthcare/ [Accessed 30/11/19].

NHS England (2019). *Statistical Press Notice: Monthly Delayed Transfers of Care Data, England, March 2019*. Available at: https://www.england.nhs.uk/statistics/statistical-work-areas/delayed-transfers-of-care/statistical-work-areas-delayed-transfers-of-care-delayed-transfers-of-care-data-2018-19/ [Accessed 9/5/19].

Nilsson, D., Joubert, L., Holland, L. and Posenelli, S. (2013). 'The Why of Practice: Using PIE to Analyse Social Work Practice in Australian Hospitals', *Social Work in Health Care* 52(2–3), pp. 280–295.

Nugus, P., Greenfield, D., Travaglia, J., Westbrook, J. and Braithwaite, J. (2010). 'How and Where Clinicians Exercise Power: Interprofessional Relations in Health Care', *Social Science and Medicine,* 71(5), pp. 898–909.

O'Malia, A., Hills, A.P. and Wagner, S. (2014). 'Repositioning Social Work in the Modern Workforce: The Development of a Social Work Assistant Role', *Australian Social Work,* 67(4). pp. 593–603.

Office for National Statistics (2015). *National Population Projections.* London: Office for National Statistics. Available at: https://www.ons.gov.uk/peoplepopulationandcommunity/populationandmigration/populationprojections/compendium/nationalpopulationprojections/2015-10-29/summaryresults [Accessed 28/7/17].

Office for National Statistics (2018). *Overview of the UK Population: November 2018.* London: Office for National Statistics. Available at: https://www.ons.gov.uk/peoplepopulationandcommunity/populationandmigration/populationestimates/articles/overviewoftheukpopulation/november2018 [Accessed 10/11/19].

Olsen, J.M. (2014). 'Health Coaching: A Concept Analysis', *Nursing Forum,* 49(1), pp. 18–29.

Osborn, H. (1996). 'One Door – Many Mansions: 1974–1995', in J. Baraclough, G. Dedman, H. Osborn and P. Willmott (eds.), *100 Years of Health Related Social Work.* Birmingham, UK: BASW.

Owens, J.M. and Garbe, R.A. (2015). 'Effect of Enhanced Psychosocial Assessment on Readmissions of Patients with Chronic Obstructive Pulmonary Disease', *Social Work in Health Care,* 54(3). pp. 234–251.

Oxford Centre for Evidence-based Medicine (2011). *Levels of Evidence Table.* Oxford: Oxford Centre for Evidence-based Medicine. Available at: http://www.cebm.net/mod_product/design/files/CEBM-Levels-of-Evidence-2.1.pdf [Accessed 10/7/13].

Palmer, S., Tubbs, I. and Whybrow, A. (2003). 'Health Coaching to Facilitate the Promotion of Healthy Behaviour and Achievement of Health-related Goals', *International Journal of Health Promotion and Education,* 41(3), pp. 91–93.

Parry, N. and Parry, J. (1979). 'Social Work, Professionalism and the State', in N. Parry, M. Rustin and C. Satyamurti (eds.), *Social Work, Welfare and the State.* London, UK: Edward Arnold.

Payne, G. and Williams, M. (2005). 'Generalization in Qualitative Research', *Sociology,* 39(2), pp. 295–314.

Payne, M. (2000). *Anti-bureaucratic Social Work.* Birmingham, UK: Venture Press.

Payne, M. (2002). 'The Role and Achievements of a Professional Association in the Late Twentieth Century: The British Association of Social Workers 1970–2000', *British Journal of Social Work,* 32, 969–995.

Payne, M. (2005). *The Origins of Social Work: Continuity and Change.* Basingstoke, UK: Palgrave Macmillan.

Payne, M. (2012). *Citizenship Social Work with Older People.* Bristol, UK: Policy Press.

Payne, M. (2014). *Modern Social Work Theory.* 4th Edition. Basingstoke, UK: Palgrave Macmillan.

Penna, S. and O'Brien, M. (2013). 'Neoliberalism', in M. Gray and S.A. Webb (eds.), *Social Work Theories and Methods.* 2nd Edition. London, UK: Sage.

Petersén, A.C. and Olsson, J.I. (2015). 'Calling Evidence-Based Practice into Question: Acknowledging Phronetic Knowledge in Social Work', *British Journal of Social Work*, 45(5). pp. 1581–1597.

Phillips, J. and Waterson, J. (2005). 'Care Management and Social Work: A Case Study of the Role of Social Work in Hospital Discharge to Residential or Nursing Home Care', *European Journal of Social Work*, 5(2), pp. 171–186.

Phillips, J., Walford, N. and Hockey, A. (2011). 'How Do Unfamiliar Environments Convey Meaning to Older People?', *International Journal of Ageing and Later Life*, 6(2), pp. 73–102.

Phillips, J., Dobbs, C., Burholt, V. and Marston, H. (2015). 'Extracare: Does It Promote Resident Satisfaction Compared to Residential and Home Care?', *British Journal of Social Work*, 45(3), pp. 949–967.

Phillipson, C. (2013). *Ageing*. Cambridge, UK: Polity.

Phillipson, C. and Walker, A. (1987). 'The Case for a Critical Gerontology', in S. Di Gregorio (ed.), *Social Gerontology: New Directions*. London: Croom Helm.

Phoenix, J. (1999). *Making Sense of Prostitution*. Basingstoke, UK: Palgrave.

Pickard, S. (2016). *Age Studies*. London, UK: Sage.

Pithouse, A. (1987). *Social Work: The Social Organization of an Invisible Trade*. Aldershot, UK: Avebury.

Plafky, C.S. (2016). 'From Neuroscientific Research Findings to Social Work Practice: A Critical Description of the Knowledge Utilisation Process', *British Journal of Social Work*, 46(6), pp. 1502–1519.

Plank, A., Mazzoni, V. and Cavada, L. (2012). 'Becoming a Caregiver: New Family Carers' Experience During the Transition from Hospital to Home', *Journal of Clinical Nursing*, 21(13–14), pp. 2072–2082.

Plath, D. (2014). 'Implementing EBP: An Organisational Perspective', *British Journal of Social Work*, 44(4), pp. 905–923.

Pockett, R. (2002). 'Staying in Hospital Social Work', *Social Work in Health Care*, 36 (1), pp. 1–24.

Porter, R. (1999). *The Greatest Benefit to Mankind: A Medical History of Humanity*. London, UK: Norton.

Power, M. (1997), *The Audit Society: Rituals of Verification*. Oxford, UK: Oxford University Press.

Power, M. (2004). *The Risk Management of Everything: Rethinking the Politics of Uncertainty*. London, UK: DEMOS.

Public Accounts Committee (2018). *Investigation into NHS Continuing Healthcare Funding*. London: Public Accounts Committee. Available at: https://publications.parliament.uk/pa/cm201719/cmselect/cmpubacc/455/455.pdf/ [Accessed 30/11/19].

Pullen-Sansfacon, A. and Cowden, S. (2012). *The Ethical Foundations of Social Work*. Harlow, UK: Pearson.

Rachman, R. (1997). 'Hospital Social Work and Community Care', *Social Work in Health Care*, 25(1–2), pp. 211–222.

Rashid, S. (2000). 'Social Work and Professionalization: A Legacy of Ambivalence', in C. Davies, L. Finlay and A. Bullman (eds.), *Changing Practice in Health and Social Care*. London, UK: Sage.

Ray, M. and Phillips, J. (2012). *Social Work with Older People*. Basingstoke, UK: Palgrave Macmillan.

Ray, M., Bernard, M. and Phillips, J. (2009). *Critical Issues in Social Work with Older People*. Basingstoke, UK: Palgrave Macmillan.

Ray, M., Milne, A., Beech, C., Phillips, J.E., Richards, S., Sullivan, M.P., Tanner, D. and Lloyd, L. (2015). 'Gerontological Social Work: Reflections on its Role, Purpose and Value', *British Journal of Social Work*, 45(4), pp. 1296–1312.

Reay, T. and Hinings, C.R. (2005). 'The Recomposition of an Organizational Field: Health Care in Alberta', *Organization Studies*, 26(3), pp. 351–384.

Reay, T. and Hinings, C.R. (2009). 'Managing the Rivalry of Competing Institutional Logics', *Organization Studies*, 30(6), pp. 629–652.

Reinders, R.C. (1982). 'Toynbee Hall and the American Settlement Movement', *Social Service Review*, 56(1), pp. 39–54.

Richards, S., Sullivan, M.P., Tanner, D., Beech, C., Milne, A., Ray, M., Phillips, J. and Lloyd, L. (2014). 'On the Edge of a New Frontier: Is Gerontological Social Work in the UK Ready to Meet the Twenty-First-Century Challenges?', *British Journal of Social Work*, 44(8), pp. 2307–2324.

Ritzer, M. (1996). *The McDonaldization of Society*. Thousand Oaks, CA: Pine Forge Press.

Rivett, G. (1998). *From Cradle to Grave: Fifty Years of the NHS*. London, UK: King's Fund.

Rizzo, V.M. (2006). 'Social Work Support Services for Stroke Patients: Interventions and Outcomes', *Social Work in Health Care*, 43, pp. 33–56.

Rizzo, V.M. and Abrams, A. (2000). 'Utilization Review: A Powerful Social Work Role in health care settings', *Health and Social Work*, 25, pp. 264–269.

Robson, C. (1993). *Real World Research*. Oxford, UK: Blackwell.

Rockwood, K. and Mitniski, A. (2007). 'Frailty in Relation to the Accumulation of Deficits', *Journals of Gerontology Series A*, 62(7), pp. 722–727.

Rogowski, S. (2010). *Social Work: The Rise and Fall of a Profession?* Bristol, UK: Policy Press.

Rooff, M. (1972). *A Hundred Years of Family Welfare: A Study of the Family Welfare Association (formerly Charity Organisation Society) 1869–1969*. London, UK: Michael Joseph.

Rose, S.M. (1990). 'Advocacy/Empowerment: An Approach to Clinical Practice for Social Work', *Journal of Sociology and Social Welfare*, 17(2), pp. 41–51.

Rossiter, A. (2000). 'The Postmodern Feminist Condition: New Conditions for Social Work', in B. Fawcett, B. Featherstone, J. Fook and A. Rossiter (eds.), *Practice and Research in Social Work: Postmodern Feminist Perspectives*. Abingdon, UK: Routledge.

Rowlands, A. (2007). 'Medical Social Work Practice and SARS in Singapore', *Social Work in Health Care*, 45(1), pp. 57–83.

Rowntree, B.S. (1901). *Poverty: A Study of Town Life*. London, UK: Macmillan.

Rowntree, B.S. (1918). *Human Needs of Labour*. Edinburgh, UK: Nelson.

Royle, E. (2012). *Modern Britain: A Social History 1750–2010*. 3rd Edition. London: A&C Black.

Rushton, A. and Davies, P. (1984). *Social Work and Health Care*. London, UK: Heinemann.

Sackett, D.L., Rosenberg, W.M., Gray, J.H.M., Haynes, R.B. and Richardson, W.S. (1996). 'Evidence-based Practice: What It Is and What It Isn't', *British Medical Journal*, 312(7203), pp. 71–72.

Sackett, D.L., Straus, S.E., Richardson, W.S., Rosenberg, W. and Haynes, R.B. (2000). *Evidence-based medicine: How to Practice and Teach EBM*. Edinburgh, UK: Churchill Livingstone.

Sackville, A. (1986). *Hospital Almoners Association: 1903–1930*. Available at: https://www.kcl.ac.uk/scwru/swhn/2013/sackville-wp01-hospital-almoners-association-1903-to-1930.pdf [Accessed 28/11/19].

Sackville, A. (1987). *From Almoner to Medical Social Worker: 1950–1970*. Available at: http://www.kcl.ac.uk/sspp/kpi/scwru/swhn/2013/Sackville-WP04-From-Almoner-to-Medical-Social-Worker-1950-to-1970.pdf [Accessed 23/6/14].

Sackville, A. (1988a). *The Association of Psychiatric Social Workers – The Early Years*. Available at: https://www.kcl.ac.uk/sspp/policy-institute/scwru/swhn/2013/Sackville-WP06-APSW-The-Early-Years.pdf [Accessed 4/4/18].

Sackville, A. (1988b). *APSW – From Mackintosh to BASW, 1951–1970*. Available at: https://www.kcl.ac.uk/sspp/policy-institute/scwru/swhn/2013/Sackville-WP08-APSW-From-Mackintosh-to-BASW-1951-1970.pdf [Accessed 4/4/18].

Sackville, A. (1989). 'Thomas William Cramp, Almoner: The Forgotten Man in a Female Occupation', *British Journal of Social Work*, 19, pp. 95–110.

Salsberg, E., Quigley, L., Acquaviva, K., Wyche, K. and Sliwa, S. (2018). *New Social Workers: Results of the Nationwide Survey of 2017 Social Work Graduates*. Washington, DC: The George Washington University Health Workforce Institute. Available at: https://www.socialworkers.org/LinkClick.aspx?fileticket=C0r5P1zkMbQ%3D&portalid=0 [Accessed 1/8/19].

Scambler, G. (2009). 'Sociology in Medical Education', in C. Brosnan and B.S. Turner (eds.), *Handbook of the Sociology of Medical Education*. Abingdon, UK: Routledge.

Scourfield, J. (2003). *Gender and Child Protection*. Basingstoke, UK: Palgrave Macmillan.

Seebohm Report (1968). *Report of the Committee on Local Authority and Allied Personal Social Services*. London, UK: HSMO.

Seed, P. (1973). *The Expansion of Social Work in Britain*. London, UK: Routledge and Kegan Paul.

Shapiro, M., Setterlund, D., Warburton, J., O'Connor, I. and Cumming, S. (2009). 'The Outcomes Research Project: An Exploration of Customary Practice in Australian Health Settings', *British Journal of Social Work*, 39(2), pp. 318–333.

Shaw, I. (2008). 'Merely Experts? Reflections on the History of Social Work, Science and Research', *Research, Policy and Planning*, 26, pp. 57–65.

Sheldon, B. (2001), 'The Validity of Evidence-based Practice in Social Work: A Reply to Stephen Webb', *British Journal of Social Work*, 31, pp. 801–809.

Sheldon, B. and MacDonald, G. (2008). *A Textbook of Social Work*. London, UK: Routledge.

Sheldon, B., Chivers, R., Ellis, A., Mosely, A. and Tierney, S. (2005). 'A Pre-post Empirical Study of the Obstacles to, and Opportunities for, Evidence-based Practice in Social Care', in A. Bilson (ed.), *Evidence-based Practice in Social Work*. London, UK: Whiting and Birch.

Simmons, A. (2005). *A Profession and its Roots: The Lady Almoners*. London, UK: Michelangelo Press.

Simpson, G., Pfeiffer, D., Keogh, S. and Lane, B. (2016). 'Describing an Early Social Work Intervention Program for Families after Severe Traumatic Brain Injury', *Journal of Social Work in Disability and Rehabilitation*, 15(3–4), pp. 213–233.

Sims-Gold, J., Byrne, K., Hicks, E., Franke, T. and Stolee, P. (2015). '"When Things Are Really Complicated We Call the Social Worker": Post Hip-Fracture Care Transitions for Older People', *Health Social Work*, 40(4), pp. 257–265.

Skillbeck, J.K., Arthur, A. and Seymour, J. (2018). 'Making Sense of Frailty: An Ethnographic Study of the Experience of Older People Living with Complex Health Problems', *International Journal of Older People Nursing*, 13(1), e12172.

Sosin, M. and Caulum, S. (1983). 'Advocacy: A Conceptualization for Social Work Practice', *Social Work*, 28(1), pp. 12–17.

Standing, G. (2010). *The Precariat: The New and Dangerous Class*. London, UK: Bloomsbury.

Statham, J., Cameron, C. and Mooney, A. (2006). *The Tasks and Roles of Social Workers: A Focused Overview of Research Evidence*. Available at: http://discovery.ucl.ac.uk/1507248/1/Tasks_and_roles_of_social_workers_-_report.pdf [Accessed 28/3/18].

Stevenson, O. (1977). *Ageing: A Professional Perspective*. London, UK: Age Concern.

Stevenson, O. (2005). 'Genericism and Specialization: The Story Since 1970', *British Journal of Social Work*, 35(5), pp. 569–586.

Strauss, A.L., Schatzman, L., Ehrlich, D., Bucher, R. and Sabshin, M. (1963). 'The Hospital and its Negotiated Order', in E. Freidson (ed.), *The Hospital in Modern Society*. New York, NY: Free Press.

Sullivan, M.P. (2009). 'Social Workers in Community Care Practice: Ideologies and interactions with older people', *British Journal of Social Work*, 39(6), pp. 1306–1325.

Tadd, W., Hillman, A., Calnan, S., Calnan, M., Bayer, A.J. and Read, S.M. (2011). 'Right Place – Wrong Person: Dignity in the Acute Care of Older People', *Quality in Ageing and Older Adults*, 12(1), pp. 33–43.

Tannen, D. and Wallat, C. (1987). 'Interactive Frames and Knowledge Schemas in Interaction: Examples from a Medical Examination/Interview', *Social Psychology Quarterly*, 50(2), pp. 205–216.

Tanner, D. (2013). 'Identity, Selfhood and Dementia: Messages for Social Work', *European Journal of Social Work*, 16(2), pp. 155–170.

Tanner, D., Glasby, J. and McIver, S. (2015). 'Understanding and Improving Older People's Experiences of Service Transitions: Implications for Social Work', *British Journal of Social Work*, 45(7), pp. 2056–2071.

Taylor, C. and White, S. (2000). *Practising Reflexivity in Health and Welfare: Making Knowledge*. Buckingham, UK: Open University Press.

Tennier, L.D. (1997). 'Discharge Planning: An Examination of the Perceptions and Recommendations for Improved Discharge Planning at the Montreal General Hospital', *Social Work in Health Care*, 26, pp. 41–60.

Thompson, N. (2010). *Theorizing Social Work Practice*. Basingstoke, UK: Palgrave Macmillan.

Thompson, N. (2015). *Understanding Social Work: Preparing for Practice*. 4th Edition. Basingstoke, UK: Palgrave Macmillan.

Thompson, N. (2016). *Anti-discriminatory Practice*. 6th Edition. Basingstoke, UK: Palgrave Macmillan.

Todd Report (1968). *Report of the Royal Commission on Medical Education 1965–68*. London, UK: HMSO.

Trevithick, P. (2012). *Social Work Skills and Knowledge: A Practice Handbook*. 3rd Edition. Maidenhead, UK: McGraw-Hill/Open University Press.

Van Heugten, K. (2011). *Social Work Under Pressure: How to Overcome Stress, Fatigue and Burnout in the Workplace*. London, UK: Jessica Kingsley.

Waddington, K. (2011). *An Introduction to the Social History of Medicine*. Basingstoke, UK: Palgrave Macmillan.

Walker, A. (2012). 'The New Ageism', *Political Quarterly*, 83(4), pp. 812–819.

Wallace, J. and Pease, B. (2011). 'Neoliberalism and Australian Social Work: Accommodation or resistance?', *Journal of Social Work*, 11(2), pp. 132–142.

Walter, I., Nutley, S., Percy-Smith, J., McNeish, D. and Frost, S. (2004). *SCIE Knowledge Review 7: Improving the Use of Research in Social Care*. London, UK: SCIE.

Wastell, D. and White, S. (2012). 'Blinded by Neuroscience: Social Policy, the Family and the Infant Brain', *Families, Relationships and Societies*, 1(3), pp. 397–414.

Wastell, D. and White, S. (2017). *Blinded by Science: The Social Implications of Epigenetics and Neuroscience*. Bristol, UK: Policy Press.

Wastell, D., White, S., Broadhurst, K., Peckover, S. and Pithouse, A. (2010). 'Children's Services in the Iron Cage of Performance Management: Street-level Bureaucracy and the Spectre of Svejkism', *International Journal of Social Welfare*, 19(3), pp. 310–320.

Webb, S.A. (2007). 'The Comfort of Strangers: Social Work, Modernity and Late Victorian England – Part I', *European Journal of Social Work*, 10, pp. 39–54.

Webb, S.A. (2001). 'Some Considerations on the Validity of Evidence-based Practice in Social Work', *British Journal of Social Work*, 31(1), pp. 51–79.

Weber, M. ([1922]2015). *Weber's Rationalism and Modern Society*. Trans. T. Waters and D. Waters. New York, NY: Palgrave Macmillan.

Welsh Government (2015). *Social Services and Well-being (Wales). Act 2014 Part 3 Code of Practice (assessing the needs of individuals)*. Available at: https://gov.wales/sites/default/files/publications/2019-05/part-3-code-of-practice-assessing-the-needs-of-individuals.pdf [Accessed 1/11/19].

Westbrook, J.I., Duffield, C., Li, L. and Creswick, N.J. (2011). 'How Much Time Do Nurses Have for Patients? A Longitudinal Study Quantifying Hospital Nurses' Patterns of Task Time Distribution and Interactions with Health Professionals', *BMC Health Services Research*, 11(1), 319.

White, P., Hillman, A. and Latimer, J. E. (2012). 'Ordering, Enrolling, and Dismissing: Moments of Access Across Hospital Spaces', *Space and Culture*, 15(1), pp. 68–87.

Willis, E. (1989). *Medical Dominance*. Revised Edition. Sydney, Australia: Allen and Unwin.

Willmott, P. (1996). '1895–1945: The First 50 Years', in J. Baraclough, G. Dedman, H. Osborn and P. Willmott (eds.), *100 Years of Health Related Social Work*. Birmingham, UK: BASW.

Wilson, K., Ruch, G., Lymbery, M. and Cooper, A. (2011). *Social Work: An Introduction to Contemporary Practice*. 2nd Edition. Harlow, UK: Pearson Longman.

Windle, K., Wagland, R., Forder, J., D'Amico, F., Janssen, D. and Wistow, G. (2009). *National Evaluation of Partnerships for Older People Projects: Final Report*. Canterbury, UK: Personal Social Services Research Unit, University of Kent.

Witkin, S.L. (1996). 'If Empirical Practice is the Answer, Then What is the Question?', *Social Work Research*, 20(2), pp. 69–75.

Witkin, S.L. (2017). *Transforming Social Work: Social Constructionist Reflections on Contemporary and Enduring Ideas*. Basingstoke, UK: Palgrave Macmillan.

Yam, B.M. (2004). 'From Vocation to Profession: The Quest for Professionalization of Nursing', *British Journal of Nursing*, 13(16), pp. 978–982.

Index

Abbott, A. 103
Abortion Act 1967 28
abuse 52, 70, 83, 91
active ageing 13–14,
advocacy: for CHC 107–108, 110–111;
    definition and meaning 79–80, 90, 94;
    independent 95; limitations of 94, 117;
    as part of discharge planning 9, 37–40,
    44, 90–96, 119–121, 124
ageing population 4, 11, 31, 37,
    124–125, 127
ageism: in hospitals 6–9; in social work
    11–12; in society 14, 16, 18, 92,
    124–125
Allen, D. 103, 106
almoner 19, 22–26
Almoners' Committee 23–24
Almoners' Council 24
Alzheimer's disease see dementia
AMHP 31
anti-oppressive practice 80
approved mental health professional see
    AMHP
approved social worker see AMHP
assessment: for CHC 10, 107–110; for
    discharge planning 9, 28–31, 25–37,
    69–71, 73–74, 90–91; of means 23, 25;
    of mental capacity 10–11, 77, 84,
    109–110; as multi-disciplinary task
    103–104, 106, 111; of risk 95
Atkinson, P. 56, 58,
austerity 31–32, 88, 126 see also
    resources, scarcity of
Australia 38, 40, 125–126

backstage see frontstage//backstage
Bailey, R. 29, 66, 116
Banks, S. 82, 121
Barnett, S.A. 21

BASW 27, 30
Bauman, Z. 3, 15–18, 30, 63–68, 71, 73,
    116, 118–119, 121
bed blocking see Delayed transfer
    of care
bed flow see patient flow
Beddoe, L. 43
best interests 11, 72–73, 84
Bevan, A. 3
biomedical model 34, 95
bio-psychosocial model 44
Bradby, H. 34
Brake, M. 29, 66, 116
Brewer, C. 22–23, 27, 29
British Association of Social Workers see
    BASW
brokerage 69, 74, 94
bureaucracy: within hospital 65–68; in
    social work practice 69, 74–76, 84,
    103, 105, 115–116, 121–123; theory of
    63, 73, 121
Burns, T. 97–98

Canada 39, 40–41
cancer 16, 39, 45, 119
Cannon, I. 23
care management 14, 35, 38, 45, 120, 123
care package see package of care
care plan 73–75, 86–87, 90–92
care planning 29, 37–38, 80, 86, 120,
    126–127 see also assessment
carers see Family carers
casework 21–22, 80, 96
CBT see cognitive behavioural therapy
charity 20–21
Charity Organisation Society 20–22, 24,
    54, 80, 122
CHC see Continuing Healthcare
child protection 28–29

choice: consumer 15, 29, 36, 74; over lifestyle 82, 90–92, 94, 119, 126 *see also liquid modernity*
chronic illness 17, 125, 127
cognitive behavioural therapy 37, 39
community care 14, 35, 70, 89, 94, 121
Community Care (Delayed Discharge) Act 2003 8
complexity: health conditions 5–7, 9; social needs 64, 86, 112,
consumerism 29–31, 35
continuing healthcare: eligibility 10, 73–74; social work assessment for 10, 64, 106–110
COS *see Charity Organisation Society*
counselling *see relational work*
Court of Protection 112
Craig, S.L. 41, 43–44, 76, 102
crisis intervention 38–40
critical best practice 51–53, 124, 126
critical gerontology 11–14, 15, 80, 124–125, 127

Davies, M. 37, 123–124
Decision Supporting Tool 73
dehumanisation 65, 67, 71–74, 115–116, 121, 123
delayed transfer of care 6–9, 64, 66–68, 76, 101
dementia 14, 16–17, 75, 82, 92, 119
Denzin, N.K. 50, 61
deontology 49, 85, 87, 116
Deprivation of Liberty Safeguards 73, 94
de-professionalisation 29
dignity 6, 18, 53, 88
Dingwall, R. 107
direct payments *see personalisation*
disabled people's movement 30
disadvantage 14, 21, 79, 116, 120, 124
disagreements: family members 11, 91, 93, 112–113; interprofessional 11, 84, 93, 108–110
discharge planning: prominence in social work of 3, 28–29, 34; practices 9, 35–40, 44–46, 68–71, 123–125 *see also assessment*
discretion 57, 61, 63, 74–78, 116, 122
discrimination 14, 16, 80
doctors: practices of 4–5, 105; roles of 28, 77, 98, 102, 110; views of 105, 110
Dominelli, L. 30, 50–51, 70, 79, 86, 122
dramatisation of role 97, 98–102, 108, 112, 117

dramaturgy 98–102
Dustin, D. 29, 31, 69–70, 115, 118

efficacy 42, 50, 56, 126
efficiency 9, 67, 68–71, 74
eligibility 29, 75, 91
emancipatory social work 35, 45, 80, 90–93, 119
emotional labour 111–113
empathy 71–72, 81, 85, 94, 121
empowerment: through consumer choice 30, 35–36; as social work aim 59, 79–81, 90–96, 116–118, 123
England 4, 8, 10, 46
escalation 66–67, 76
ethics 49, 85, 87
ethnography 55, 61
European Convention on Human Rights 82, 85
evidence-based practice 41, 47–51, 56
expertise: in medical care 4, 6–7, 14, 34, 98, 110; of social worker 25, 43, 95, 104, 123

fabricated illness 67, 86–87
falls 6, 91, 120
family carers 11, 17, 103, 120
feminism 49
Ferguson, H. 51, 53, 55, 89, 96, 124
financial assessment 25
Fordism 15, 68–69, 115
Foucault, M. 13, 21, 49, 95
fourth Age 12–13, 16
frailty 13, 16, 88, 119–120
frame analysis 97–98, 102–114, 117–118, 124–125
Freidson, E. 24
frontstage/backstage 99–100, 113

Gambrill, E. 48
Gardner, A. 35, 74
Garrett, P.M. 16, 120
gender 16, 23, 31
Germany 39
gerontology *see Critical Gerontology*
Giddens, A. 15–16, 70, 87, 119
Gilleard, C. 12–13, 125
Glasby, J. 8, 42, 44
Goffman, I. 97–101, 102, 105, 107–108, 113, 117
Gorman, H. 31
Grenier, A. 12–13, 125
Griffiths Report 15, 29
grounded theory 62

Hammersley, M. 50, 61
Hastings, S.J. 11, 17
health coaching 38, 125–127
hierarchy: of professions 26, 43, 98–100, 110–111, 117–118, 121 *see also status of social work*; of evidence 47–48, 52–54
Higgs, P. 12–13, 125
Hillman, A. 6, 17, 88
Hinings, C.R. 98, 112
Hochschild, A.R. 111
holistic 6, 8, 9, 37, 44, 65, 126
holocaust, modernity and the 30, 63–68, 71–74
Hong Kong 40–41, 44
Hospital Almoners' Association 24
hospitals: institutional culture of 4–9, 34, 64–67, 98–105; management of *see managers*
Hugman, R. 25, 80
human rights 80–85, 88, 95–96, 116
Human Rights Act 1998 82

Ife, J. 79, 82, 85
Illich, I. 27
individualism 15–18, 36 *see also liquid modernity*
inequality 12, 16, 21, 66, 120
Institute of Hospital Almoners 24
institutional failings 81, 84, 88, 94, 117
instrumental rationality 63, 65
International Federation of Social Workers 79–80, 96, 116, 122–123
interprofessional *see multidisciplinary working*

Johnson, T.J. 27, 94

key performance indicator *see performance indicator*

Lait, J. 22–23, 27, 29
Larson, M.S. 27, 94
Laslett, P. 12
Latimer, J. 5, 7, 17, 41, 56, 105
life course *see life transitions*
life expectancy 4, 16, 119
life politics 15–16, 119, 121
life transitions 14, 39–40
Lincoln, Y.S. 50, 61
Lipsky, M. 57, 75–77, 116, 122
liquid modernity 3, 15–18, 32, 118–123
Lishman, J. 12, 19, 95

Local Authority Social Services Act 1970 27
Lock, C. 22
Lymbery, M. 11, 21, 25, 29–31, 35, 90, 118, 121

MacDonald, G. 47, 58
maintenance theory 123–124
management: of hospitals 6–9, 64–67, 100–101, 109, 115; of local authorities 9, 30, 64, 66–67, 74, 109, 121–122 *see also social work manager*
managerialism 29–31, 64–68, 115–116
Manchée, D.M. 24, 25
Manthorpe, J. 21
marginalisation 11, 14, 91
market in social care 29–31, 35, 94, 121
Marxism 49
maternity 23, 28
medical model *see biomedical model*
medical social worker 27
medicine: as profession 4–5, 7; development and history 4–5, 7; medical education 19, 22, 25–26; specialisation 4, 5, 7, 43
mental capacity: assessment of 10–11, 31, 77, 84, 109–110; importance in decision-making 11, 82, 89
Mental Capacity Act 2005 10, 31, 77, 84, 110
mental health 28, 31
Mental Health Act 1983 31
Mills, C.W. 124
Moberly Bell, E. 22–23
moral 48, 52
Morgan, S. 92, 117
motivational interviewing 37, 39, 125
multidisciplinary working 9, 10, 41, 43–44, 101, 103–107
Munro, E. 67, 111
Muskat, B. 41, 76, 102

neglect 70, 83, 89, 91, 95
neoliberalism 15, 17, 120–123
new public management *see managerialism*
NHS: foundation and development 3–4, 26; management *see managers*
NHS and Community Care Act 1990 28, 32
Northern Ireland 36
nurse managers *see management of hospitals*

nurses: practices of 5, 88, 92, 101, 108; roles of 5, 44–45, 76, 104, 108, 112; views of 22, 42–43, 89, 92, 104, 106–107
nursing home *see residential care*
nursing profession 5, 25, 100–102

Obama, B. 37
occupational therapy 5, 65, 76, 98, 103–104
Office for National Statistics 4, 31
oncology *see cancer*
ONS *see Office for National Statistics*
oppression 16, 50–51, 80, 116, 120, 124,

package of care 56, 64, 69, 82, 105, 115
Parkinson's disease 16, 119
patient flow 7, 8, 64–67, 87, 100, 113
Payne, M. 11, 20, 21, 27, 30–31, 54, 67, 68, 78, 81
performance indicators 8, 30, 51, 57, 67–68, 126
personal budgets *see personalisation*
personalisation 35–36, 45, 74
person-centred 43, 86
Phillips, J. 14, 17, 29, 90–91, 120, 124
Phillipson, C. 12
physiotherapy 5, 98, 103
Pickard, C. 12, 91
Pithouse, A. 55, 57
Plafky, C.S. 54, 57
Poor Law Amendment Act 1834 20
poor laws, Elizabethan 20
population demographics 4, 11, 54
Porter, R. 4, 19, 22
positivism 50, 54, 61
Postle, K. 29–31, 35
postmodernism 50
POVA 70, 83–84, 88–89, 94, 112
poverty 20–21, 23
power: of individual 13, 15, 17, 116, 119; professional 24, 32, 35, 79, 94–95, 103; relations 45, 50, 54–55, 80–81, 90–92
practice wisdom 52
practitioner researcher 58, 127
precarity 16–17,
prevention 37–39, 42, 46, 125–127
procedures 69
professionalisation of social work 19, 23–25, 27
protection of vulnerable adults *see POVA*
psychodynamic theory 21

qualifications 24, 39
quality of life *see well-being*

radical social work 21, 29, 66, 122
randomised control trial 47–48, 53
rationalisation 6, 7, 17
Ray, M. 11, 12, 14, 29, 90–91, 95, 120, 124
readmission 37–39, 42, 46, 126–127
Reay, T. 98, 112
reflective practice 53, 55
rehabilitation 10, 42, 65, 69, 88, 93
relational work 14, 28–29, 35–36, 38–39, 126
relationships, social workers and clinicians 22–23, 44, 100–102, 104–107, 111–113, 117
residential care: as discharge destination 8–9, 69, 81, 91–93, 110, 120–121; quality of 85–86, 94, 124
resources, distribution of 6, 8, 32, 73, 86–87, 127
resources, scarcity of 6–11, 31, 57, 74, 88, 125–127
risk 5–6, 38, 88, 92, 95, 117
risk-taking, positive 92, 117, 120
Ritzer, M. 30
Rogowski, S. 11, 17, 30, 79, 86, 96
role distance 113
routinisation 30, 69, 71, 74, 77
Rowntree, S. 54
Royal Free Hospital 22–23

Sackett, D.L. 47
Sackville, A. 23–24, 26
SARS 40–41
Saudi Arabia 39
Scotland 10, 36
Seebohm Report 26–27
self-determination 82–83, 89–94, 116–119, 122
service user movements 35
settlement movement 21, 80, 123
Sheldon, B. 47, 48, 57–58
social administration 21–22, 25–26, 28, 35, 38, 40
social disadvantage *see disadvantage*
social gerontology *see critical gerontology*
social justice 14, 80–81, 85–89, 95–96, 123–125
Social Services and Well-being (Wales) Act 2015 36

social work agencies *see social work organisations*
social work education 11, 23–24, 39
social work knowledge base 39, 45, 47–48, 54–56, 104, 125
social work manager 30, 57, 59, 70
social work organisations 27–28, 54–57
social work skills 39–42, 52, 71–72, 123, 125
social work values 53, 55, 71, 79–81, 122, 125
solution-focused therapy 125
speech and language therapy 5, 95
status of social work 24–28, 30–31, 42–45, 84, 102, 117 *see also hierarchy of professions*
Stevenson, O. 11, 27
Stewart, M. 22–23
stigma 14, 18, 88
street-level bureaucracy 57, 75–77, 122
strengths-based 43, 125
stroke 42
structures, social 52, 54–56, 85, 95–96, 120, 122–124
Sullivan, M.P. 14, 28, 118
surveillance 21
Sweden 39, 45
systems theory 39–40, 125

tacit knowledge 52
Taylorism 68–70, 115
therapeutic social work: approaches 12, 21, 37–40, 125–127; barriers to 28, 35, 45, 71–72
third Age 12
Thompson, N. 49, 53, 80–81, 122
time pressure: experiences of 12, 21, 37–40, 65– 68, 125–127; management of 12, 21, 37–40, 70, 125–127
Todd Report 26
training *see social work education*
transitions of care *see discharge planning*

unqualified workers 38
USA 23, 37–39, 41–42, 45, 51

Waddington, K. 19, 34
Wales 36
Wastell, D. 54–55, 67
Webb, S.A. 20, 50
Weber, M. 63, 68, 121
well-being 12, 115
what works 49–51, 126
White, S. 54–55, 62
Wilson, K. 19, 70, 77
Witkin, S. 50, 52

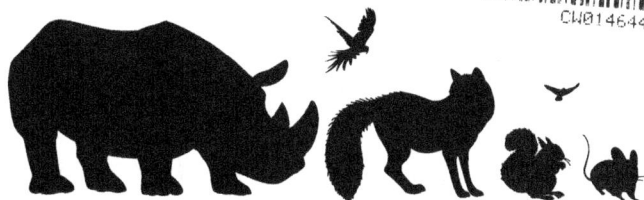

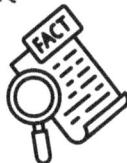

Welcome to the "Did you know?" Series - ANIMAL EDITION

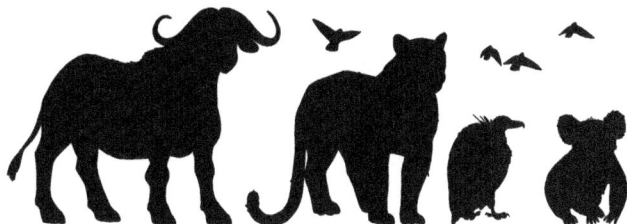

#1 Did you know? That the slowest fish in the world is actually a SeaHorse!

The Dwarf Seahorse - has a top speed of around 5 feet (1.5 metres) per hour....that's pretty slow!

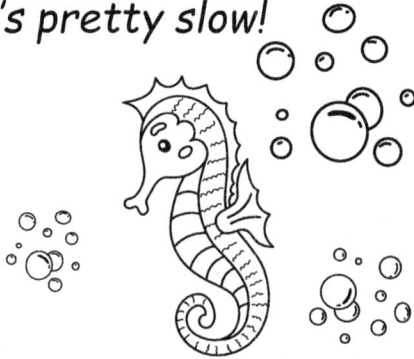

#2 Did you know? Goats have rectangular pupils!

The shape of an animals pupil is related to whether its a predator or prey, so grazing animals like goats (and sheep) have horizontal pupils to help them see danger approaching!

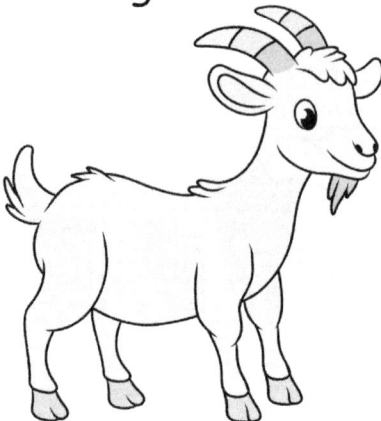

I've got my rectangular eye on you!!

#3 Did you know? That a Chameleons tongue is longer than its body!

Yep, although they are well known for their ability to change colour for camouflage, they also have another cool feature which is their tongues are typically 1.5 - 2 times their body length! This helps them catch their prey from a distance.

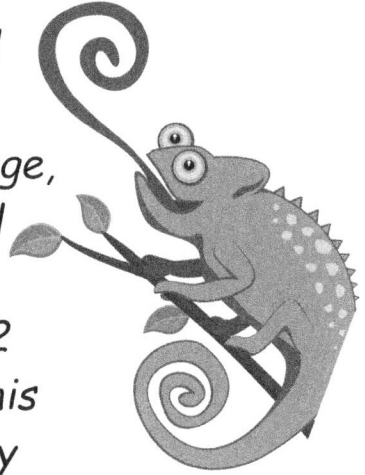

#4 Did you know? That Octopuses have 3 hearts!

1 heart pumps blood around the body and the other 2 hearts pump blood to their gills. Also Octopuses have 9 brains - 1 central brain & 1 in each of its legs!!

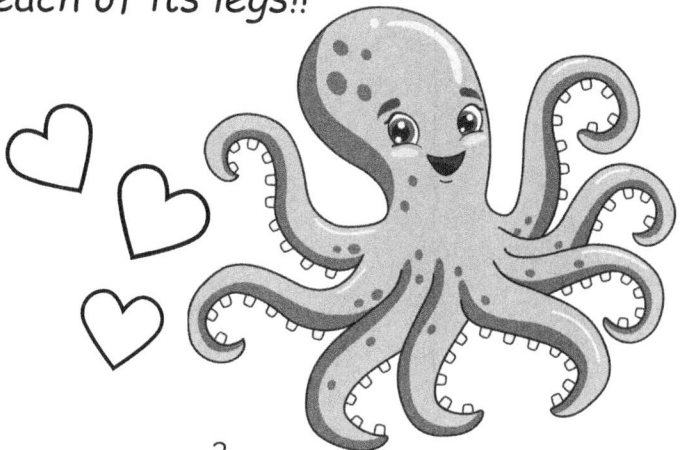

#5 Did you know? Elephants cannot jump!
Understandably really, considering they are
the largest land mammal in the world! What is
cool is, despite their bulky size they are
excellent swimmers, maybe because their
trunk is like a built in snorkel! Yet they are the
only land mammals who cannot jump!

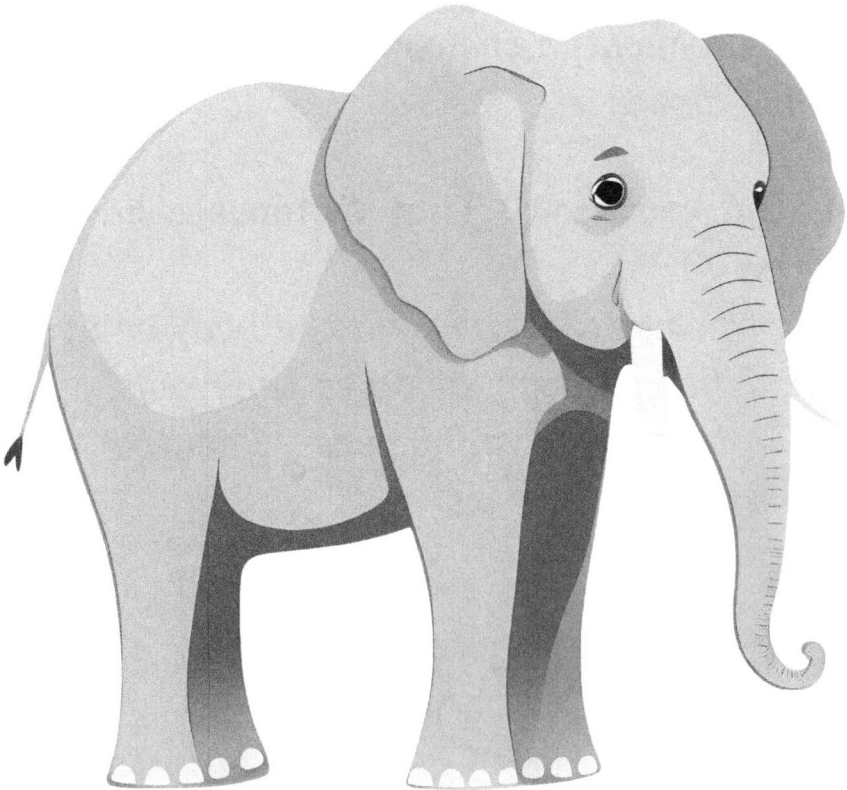

#6 Did you know? A Koala sleeps for up to 22 hours a day! *They sleep between 18-22 hours every day. This is because they have very little energy due their diet of eucalyptus leaves which are actually toxic! Whilst koalas sleep, their tummy works on digesting their food.*

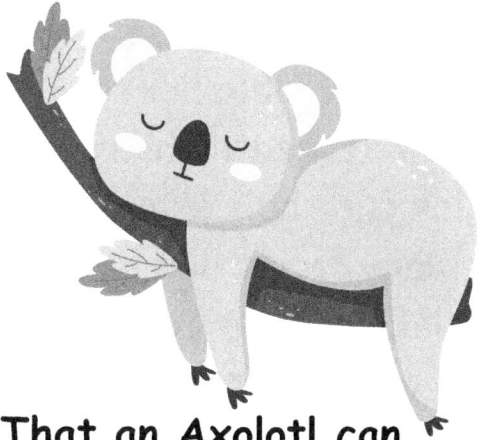

#7 Did you know? That an Axolotl can regrow its limbs!
How Freaky!! If they lose their leg or even their tail, they have the ability to simply regenerate the missing limbs. They can even regenerate parts of their brain. This is an axolotls superpower!

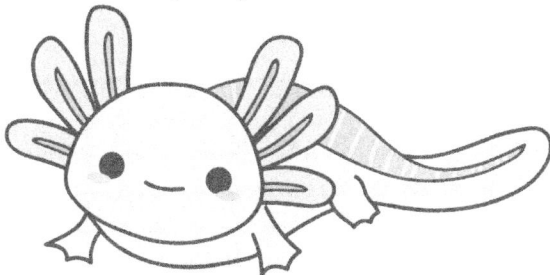

#8 Did you know? A Polar bears fur is not white!
Nope, their fur is actually transparent (see through) it only looks white because it reflects visible light and underneath their thick fur their skin is actually black. how cool! Polar bears are also great swimmers, they can swim up to 6 miles per hour and swim for long periods of time.

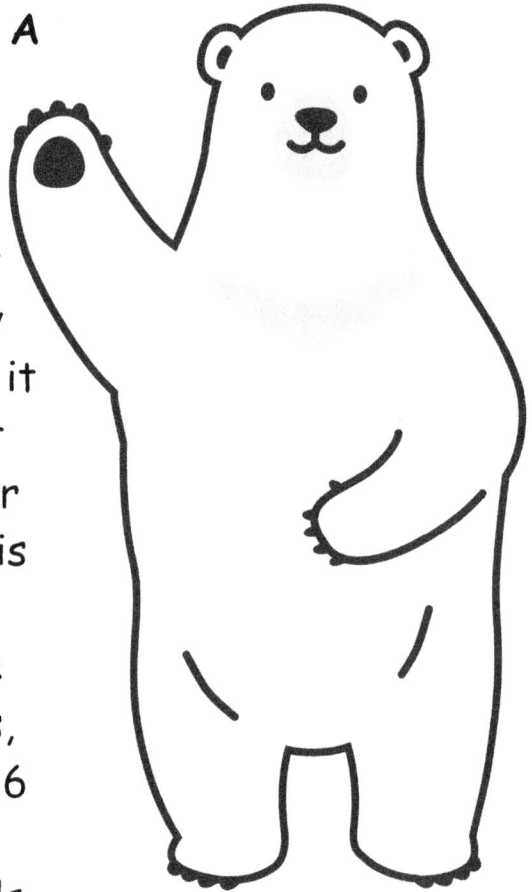

#9 Did you know? That a Woodpeckers tongue is so long it wraps around its brain!
As their tongue is so long it is tucked away by wrapping around the back of its skull. This helps protect the brain when pecking, acting like a shock absorber!

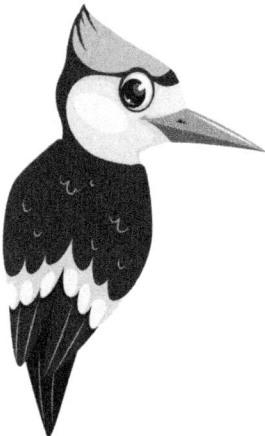

#10 Did you know? A Grizzly Bear can crush a bowling ball!

With a powerful jaw strength of around 1160 PSI (pounds per square inch) they could bite through a bowling ball. Despite this impressive fact, the polar bear actually has the strongest bite force of all bears, at 1200 PSI whereas the average human bite force is between just 120-160 PSI!

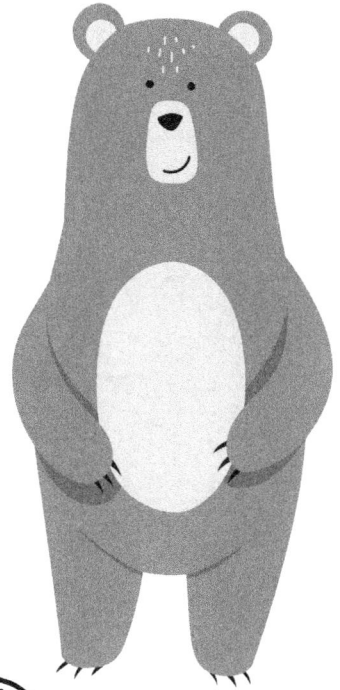

#11   Did you know? That Cows have different 'moo' accents!

Studies have shown that cows 'moo' differently depending on where they are located, so effectively cows can have regional accents!

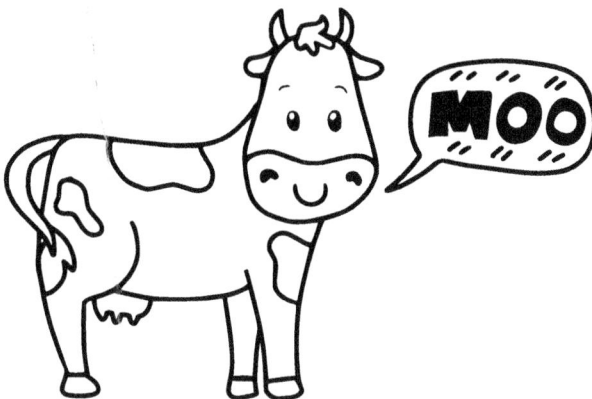

MOO

#12 Did you know? That if you shaved a Tiger you would still see their stripes!
All tigers have striped fur but their skin is also striped too. Each tiger has a striped pattern that is completely unique to them. These stripes act as camouflage, helping them blend into their surroundings whilst hunting.

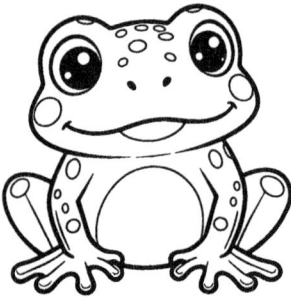

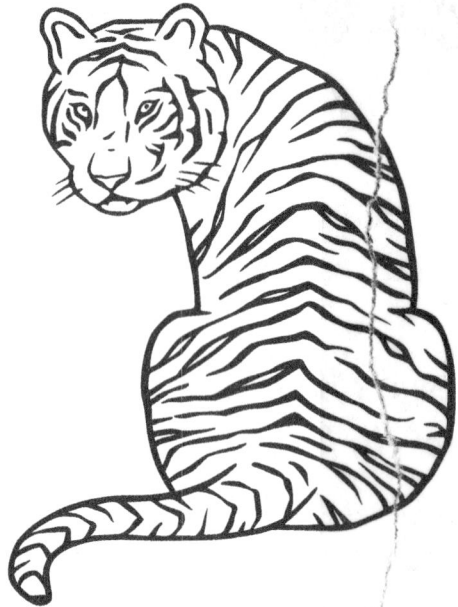

#13 Did you know? That Frogs can freeze solid and stay alive!
Species like the wood frog, can survive being frozen solid during the cold winter months and then thaw out when temperatures rise again. Other species survive by hibernating underground or under logs.

#14 Did you know? Sloths poop just once a week! *Everything in the life of a sloth is slow, including their digestive system. Due to their simple diet and slow metabolism, they only need to poop every 7-10 days. So when that time comes, they make that long, slow journey from the tree canopy down to the forest floor.*

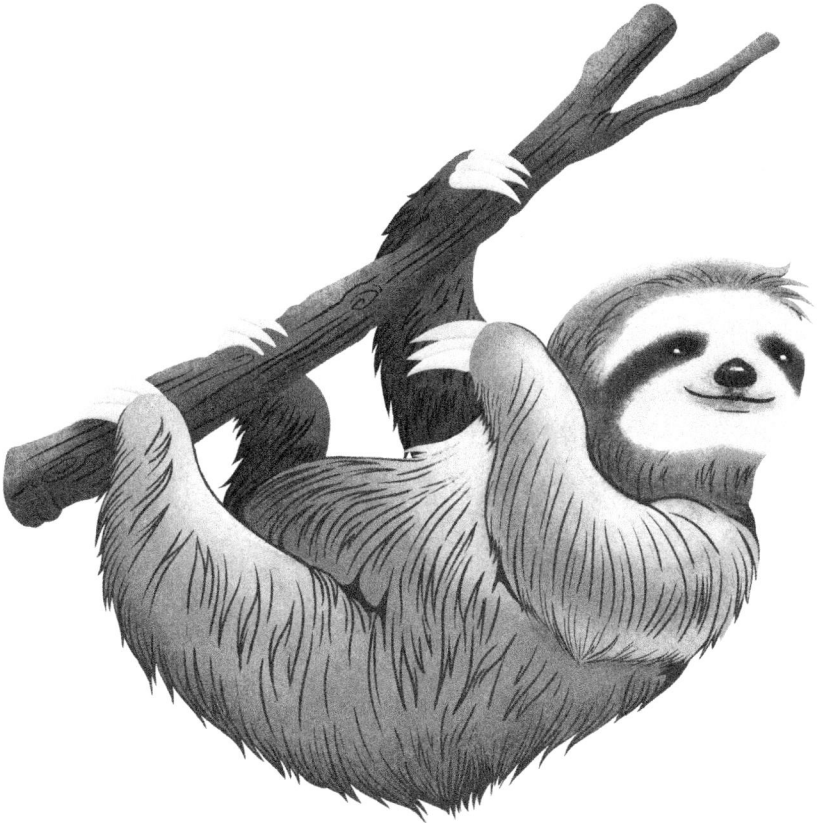

#15 Did you know?
That an Ostrich's eyes
are bigger than its
brain!

*Yes its true, but not so
surprising once you learn
that an ostrich has the
largest eyes of any land
animal! They are also the
tallest, largest, non flying
animal in the world!
Despite their size they
can run really fast, up to
a speed of 70 kilometres
per hour!*

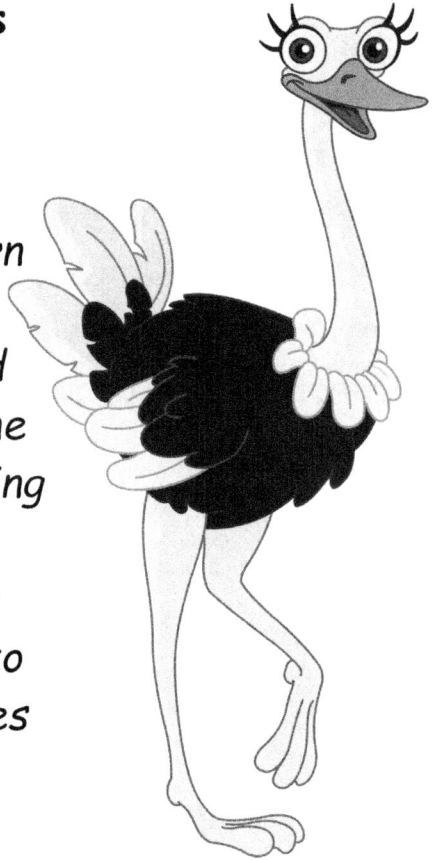

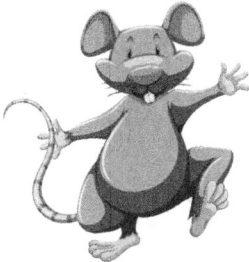

#16 Did you know? Rats laugh when
tickled!

*Studies have shown that rats make high-
pitched sounds that are similar to laughter,
when tickled. This demonstrates that rats
experience joy and happiness.*

#17 Did you know? An Electric eel can generate electric shocks that deliver up to 860 volts!

They use this shocking power to stun their prey. Standard light bulbs require around 120 volts, this means the shock of an electric eel could power a number of lightbulbs!

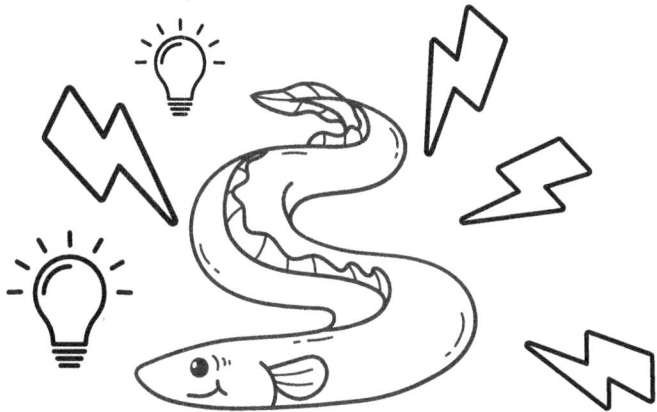

#18 Did you know? Jellyfish do not have brains or hearts!
Jellyfish do not have these important organs. They also do not have blood, bones or lungs and they breathe through the walls of their body!

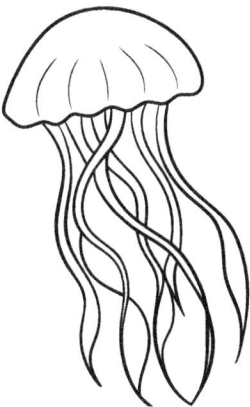

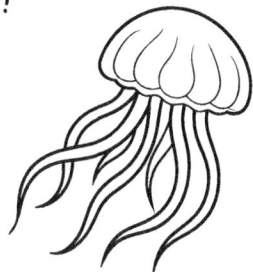

#19 Did you know? The Blue Whale's tongue weighs more than an elephant!

A blue whales tongue weighs around 3 tonnes and the average elephant weighs 2.7 tonnes so that is one giant tongue!

The blue whale is actually the largest animal on the planet, they can grow to around 90-110 feet in length! That's around the size of a Boeing 737-500 jet!!

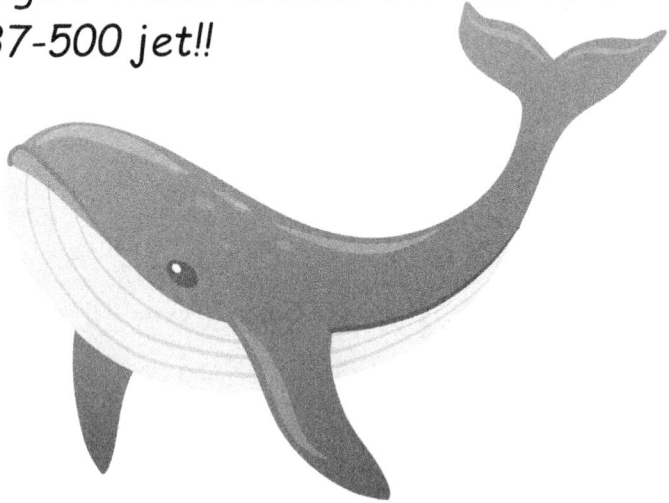

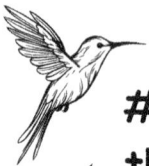

#20 Did you know? Hummingbirds are the only birds that can fly backwards!

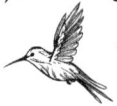

This tiny bird can fly in all directions, due to how their wings are structured. They can even fly upside down! Also, did you know that the ruby-throated hummingbird holds the record for the fastest wingbeat of any bird in the world, with 200 wingbeats per second!

#21   Did you know? That a Platypus babies are called puggles!

Platypus lay eggs like reptiles and birds but feed milk to their babies just as mammals do. Also, did you know that platypus glow under ultraviolet light. Amazing!

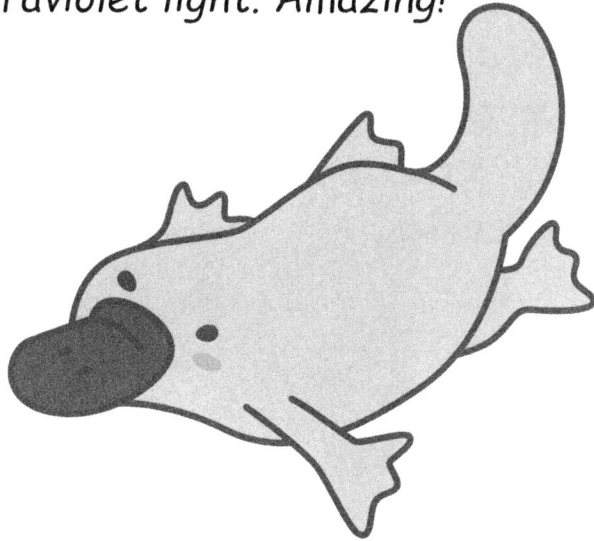

#22   Did you know? Bats are the only flying mammals in the world!

Although there are flying squirrels, they do not actually fly, they simply glide over short distances making bats the only true flying mammal.

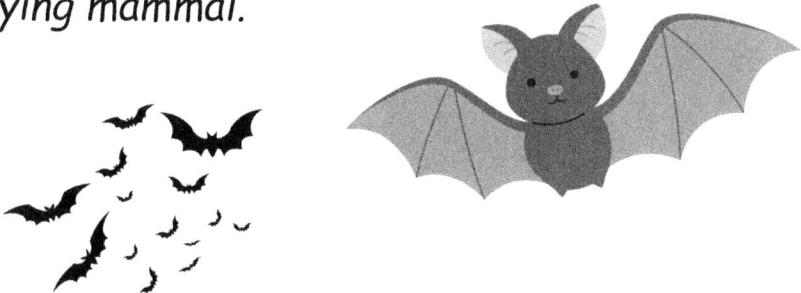

#23 Did you know? A baby Kangaroo is the size of a jellybean when born!

A baby kangaroo is called a Joey. When born, they are only an inch (2.5 centimetres) in size. At birth, not only are kangaroos incredibly small but they are also hairless and blind yet they find their way to their mothers pouch unaided. Here they will stay for a further 6-12 months depending on the species.

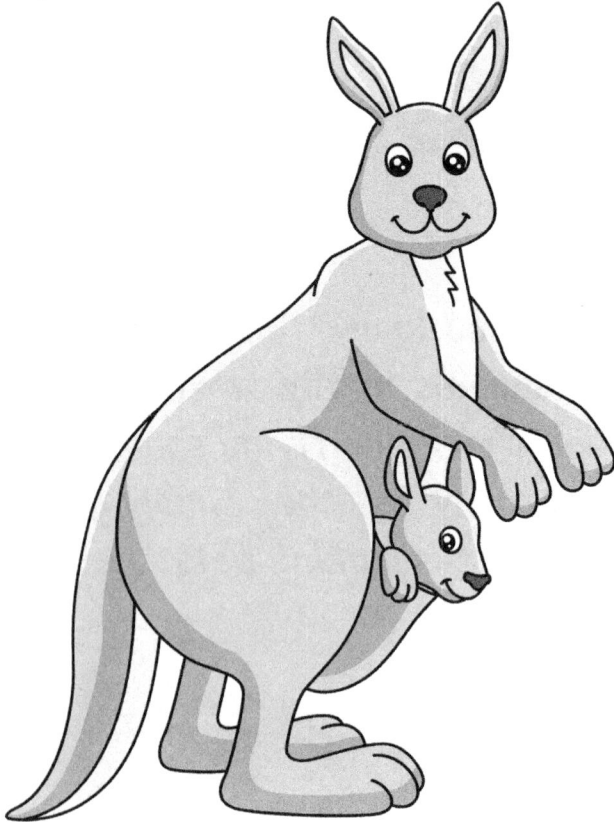

#24   Did you know? Hippos cannot swim!
Although they spend around 16 hours of the day in water, they cannot swim or float. Hippos simply sink to the bottom, due to their heavy bodies and dense bone structure. They will walk on the ground in deep water. Hippos will push off the ground and rise for air when they need to breathe.

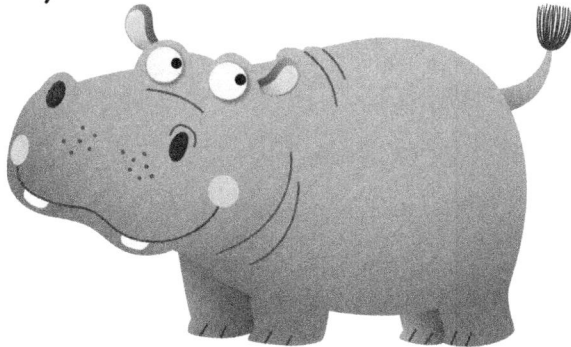

#25   Did you know? Pandas will spend over 12 hours per day eating bamboo!
Unfortunately bamboo is not very nutritious so Pandas need to eat a lot of it therefore they spend most of their day eating. Pandas can eat between 12-38 Kilograms of bamboo per day!

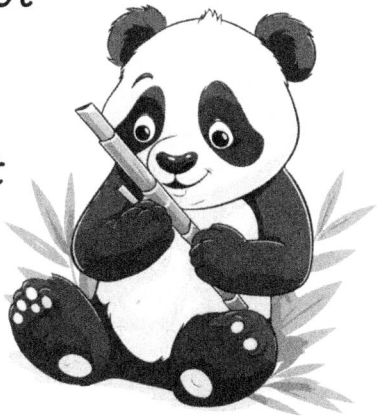

#26 Did you know? Owls don't have eyeballs!

Owls don't have eyeballs like humans, instead they have elongated eye tubes! Because of this their eyes hardly move which is why they turn their head and body to look around.

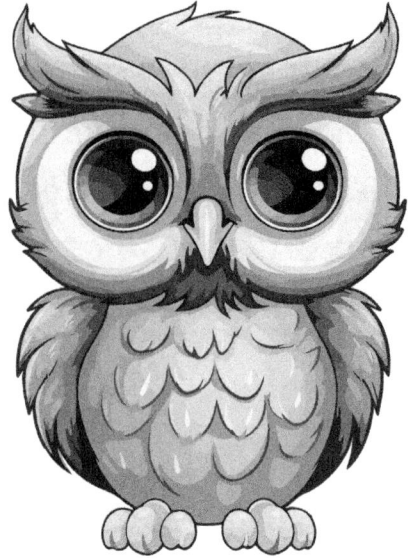

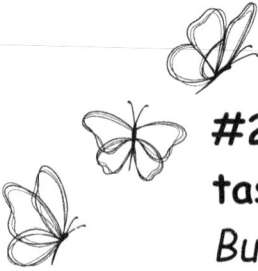

#27 Did you know? Butterflies taste with their feet!

Butterflies have receptors on their legs that help them to identify potential food. These receptors are similar to our taste buds except they are around 200 times stronger!

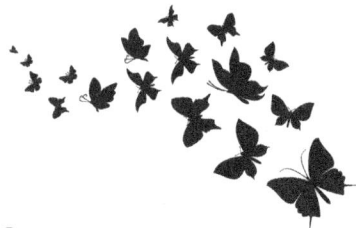

#28 Did you know? Reindeer eyes change color!

In the summer, their eyes look a golden-brown but during the winter their eyes can appear blue! This is because the reindeers eyes adapt to the darkness of winter and this helps them find food and detect predators during the longer, darker winter months. This is the only known mammal with this ability!

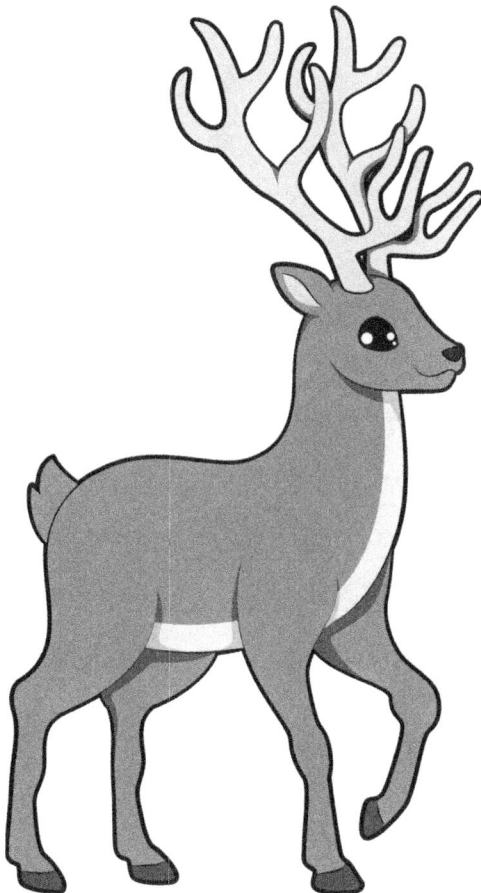

#29 Did you know? Spider silk is thinner than a strand of human hair yet 5 times stronger than steel of the same width!

It is one of the strongest natural materials in existence. Not only is it super strong but it is super flexible too. Spider silk is waterproof and can withstand temperatures from -4°C and 220°C. Pretty impressive for something that is almost 1000 times thinner than a strand of hair!

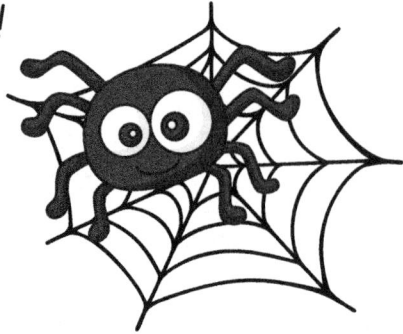

#30 Did you know? Lobsters have blue blood!

Their blood is actually colourless but when exposed to oxygen it turns blue! This is due to the presence of a copper based protein (hemocyanin). There are a few animals with blue blood including squid, octopus, snails and spiders!

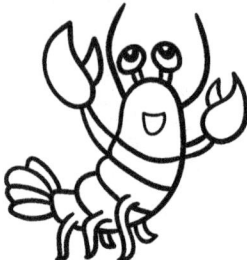

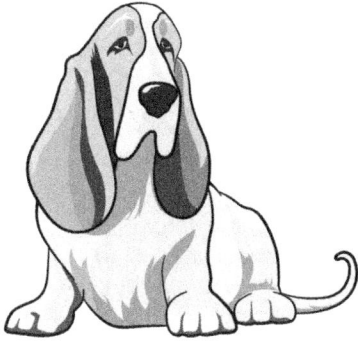

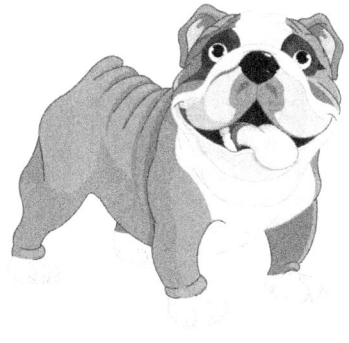

#31   Did you know? A Dogs sense of smell can be up to 100,000 times stronger than a humans!

Yes dogs have a super sense of smell. Smaller snouted (flat faced) breeds like bulldogs and pugs may not have the best sense of smell in comparison to breeds like basset hounds and beagles, breeds that were originally bred to hunt have one of the best sense of smells, yet it is believed that the Bloodhound has the ultimate sense of smell!

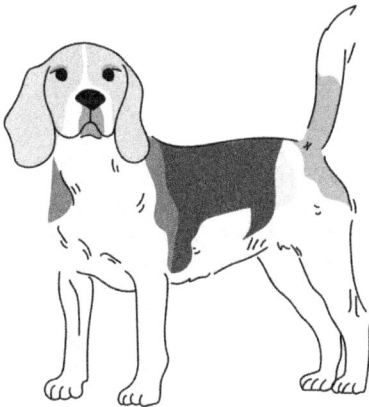

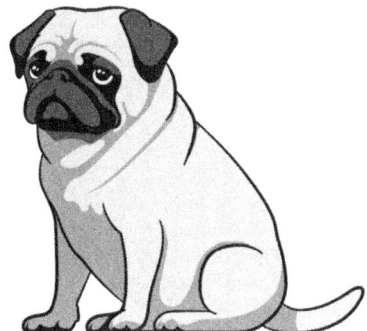

#32 Did you know? Honeybees can flap their wings 200 times per second! Because honeybee's can flap their wings so quickly it means they are able to hover and travel from flower to flower. The speed of these flapping wings is why you hear the 'buzzing' of a bee.

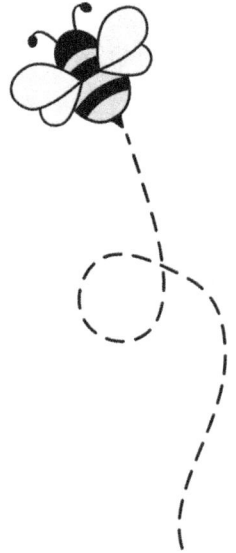

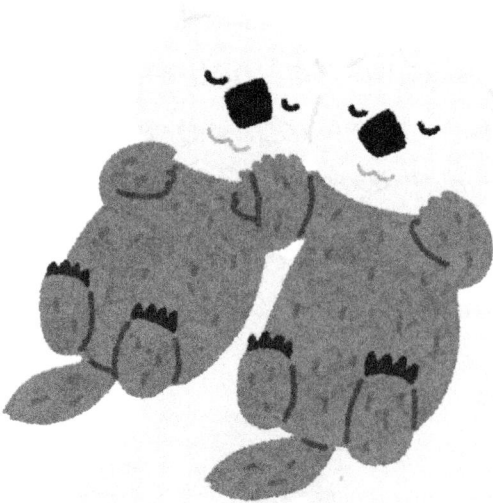

#33 Did you know? Sea Otters hold hands whilst they sleep! Sea Otters float on their backs and hold hands with their partner or family members when they sleep. This is to help avoid drifting off in the water.

#34 Did you know? Male penguins will give the gift of a pebble to a female penguin and become mates for life!

Penguins use rocks and pebbles for their nests. A male will present a pebble to the female as part of their courtship. If the female accepts this gift, the pebble will be used in the building of their nest (as rocks and pebbles are used to help keep their eggs above the surface in case of flooding). Once this is done it helps seal their bond and they mate for life! How sweet!!

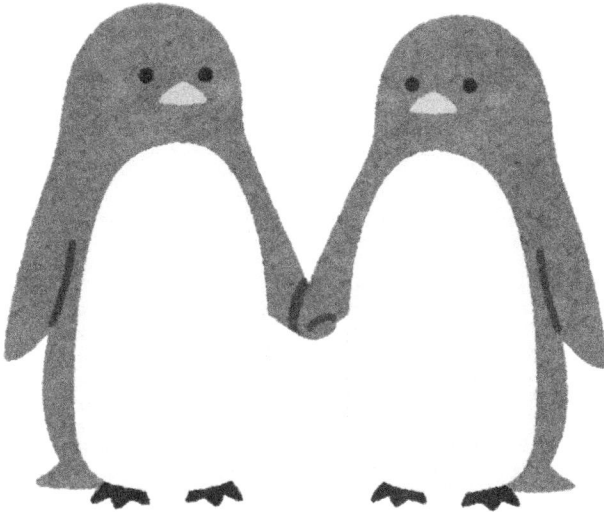

Did you know, species like the Adelie penguin have been known to happily steal pebbles and rocks from neighbouring nests to help make their own!

#35 Did you know? Dolphins will shut down half their brain whilst they sleep! This means whilst they sleep they can still keep one eye out for predators, whilst maintaining body heat. Doing this means they can also take in more oxygen from the surface water too - how clever!

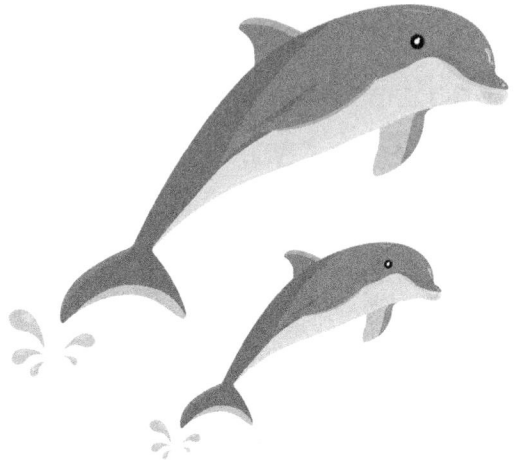

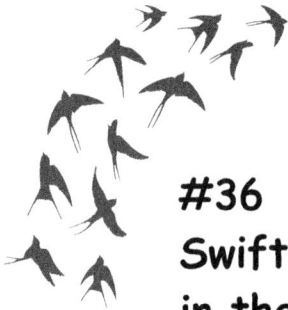

#36 Did you know? The common Swift (a migratory bird) can stay in the air for 10 whole months! These birds have one of the longest migrations in the world, travelling 14,000 miles from the UK to spend the winter in Africa! Scientists have discovered that these little birds spend 99.5% of a 10 month migration journey, completely airborne!

#37 Did you know? Turkeys roost in trees!

During the day wild turkeys spend most of their time foraging for food on the ground but during the night turkeys will sometimes roost in trees! This is more common in winter months as it helps conserve heat and helps shelter them from bad weather like wind and snow. Roosting in trees helps turkeys avoid predators too!

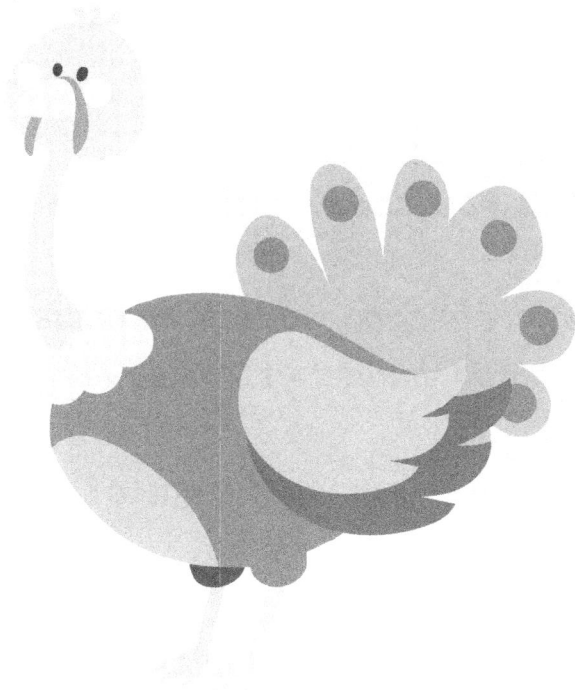

#38 Did you know? Meerkats are immune to venom!

Have you ever wondered how meerkats can eat scorpions and even some snakes, without being poisoned by a bite or sting?! That's because they have an immunity to some venoms. They will also eat fruit, vegetables, eggs, insects, lizards and obviously the poisonous scorpions and snakes too!

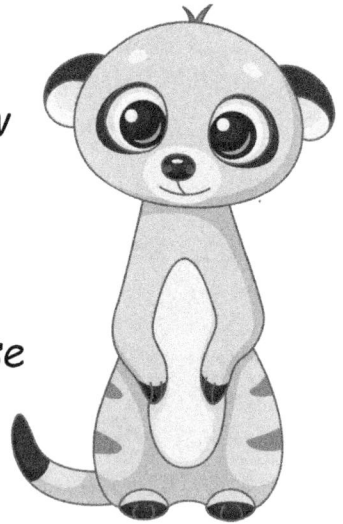

#39 Did you know? Squirrels cannot burp or vomit!

Yes, squirrels cannot burp, experience heartburn or vomit but... they can still trump (fart)!
Rats, beavers, mice and some other rodents cannot burp either!

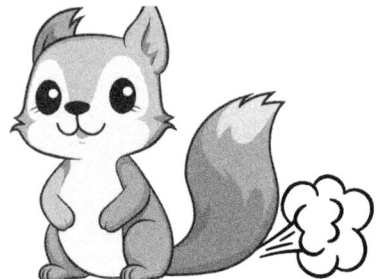

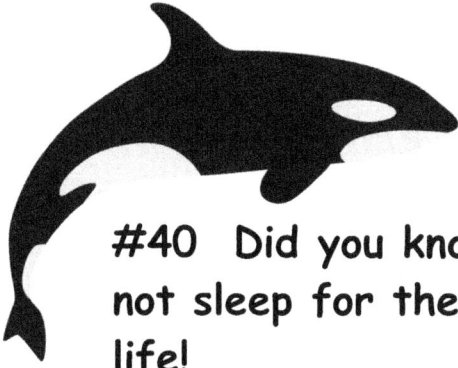

#40 Did you know? Killer Whales do not sleep for the first month of their life!

Orca (killer whales) and dolphins, do not sleep for the first month of their life...and neither do their mothers during this time either! The calves pretty much swim non stop for the first 30 days of life, this helps them to maintain body heat whilst they wait for their insulating blubber to develop. Their mother stays awake too, keeping a close eye on their offspring, teaching them to breathe, whilst looking out for predators!

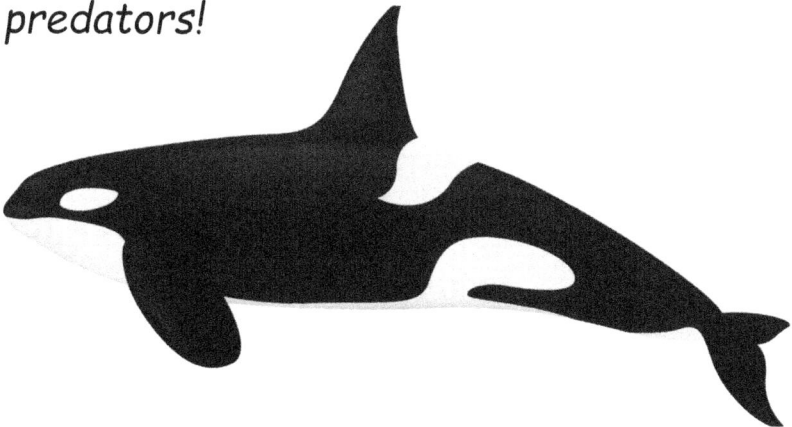

#41 Did you know? Capybaras are the worlds largest rodent!

They typically grow to 106-134cm in length, stand 50-70cm tall and typically weigh between 35-174lbs. They look like a giant guinea pig, which is actually their closest relative! Capybaras are semi-aquatic and despite their size and shape, they are skilled swimmers with the ability to hold their breath for up to 5 minutes to forage for food in water!

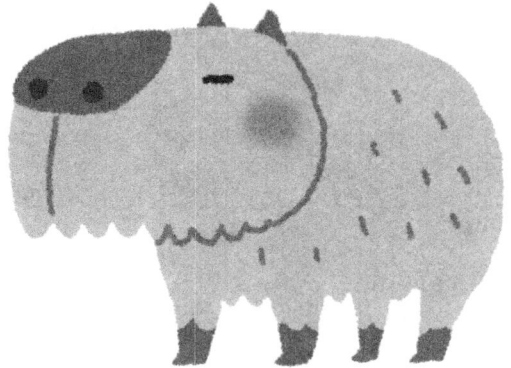

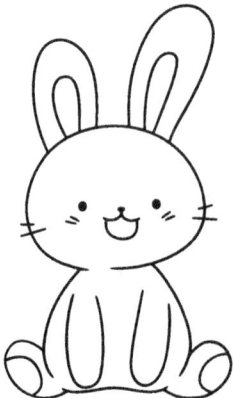

#42 Did you know? Baby rabbits are called kittens!

So kittens are not just baby cats but baby rabbits too! A male rabbit is known as a 'buck' and a female is known as a 'doe'.

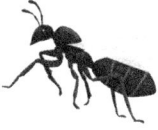

#43 Did you know? Flying Ants will chew off their own wings!
When it is time, a queen will chew off her own wings, one by one. She will then begin to dig a hole for her nest, to start a new colony.

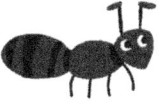

#44 Did you know? Sharks can jump out of the water and into the air!
Yes, some shark species propel their bodies into the air (mainly to catch prey) and despite their size they are able to jump out of the water! The shortfin mako shark has the best jumping abilities, jumping around 20 feet out of the water. BUT the highest jump recorded is 30 feet! This species of shark is also the fastest shark in the world!

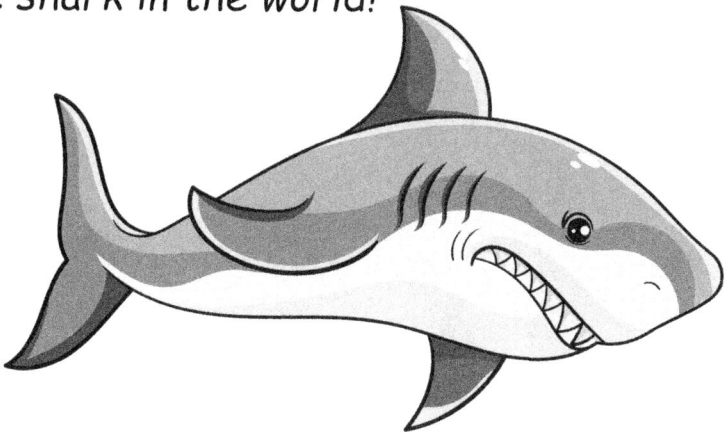

**#45 Did you know?
Flamingos are not born pink!**
*When they are born, they
hatch from their eggs and
have gray or white feathers.
They turn pink due to their
diet of algae and shrimp. Also
their bill (beak) is straight
when born but as they grow
older it begins to curve!*

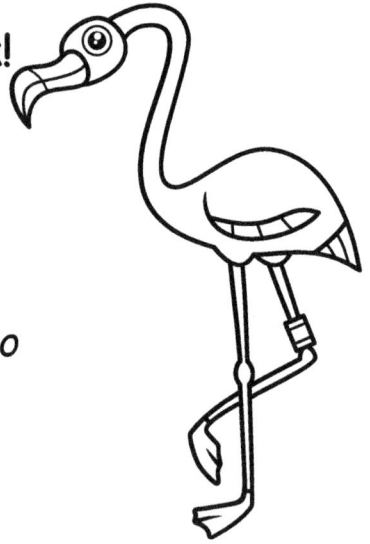

**#46 Did you know? Turtles have existed
for 220 million years!**
*Turtles belong to one of the oldest reptile
groups in the world and date back to the time
of the dinosaurs. They have one of the longest
lifespans of marine animals and the oldest
turtle (recorded) is a Seychelles giant tortoise
named Jonathan who hatched out of his egg in
1832 making him over 192 years old!*

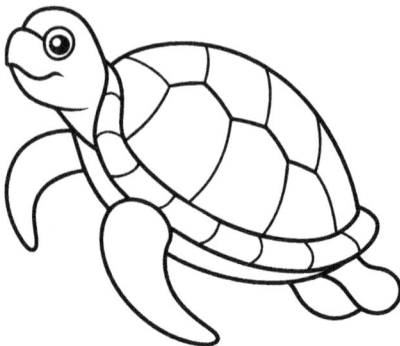

#47 Did you know? A group of Porcupines is called a prickle!
However, they do not need to live in groups thanks to their defensive spikes, so when they do gather together they are called a prickle and baby porcupines are called porcupettes!

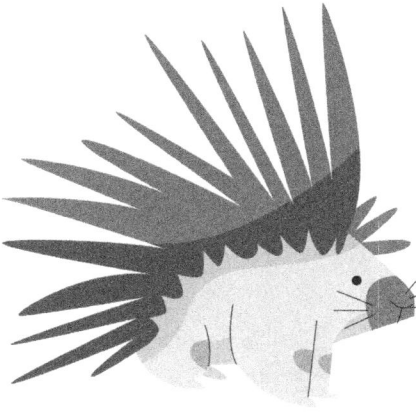

#48 Did you know? Sea Cucumbers breath through their butt!
Yes sea cucumbers are actually animals and yes they do breath through their butt....and so do some turtles too. They get their oxygen from the oxygenated water they breath in this way!

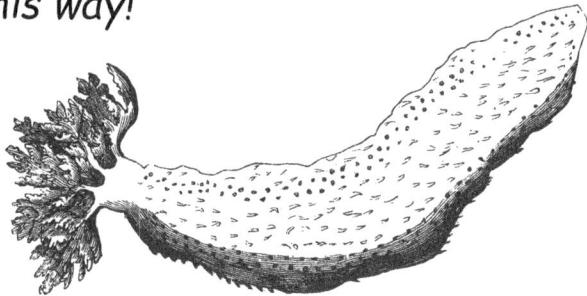

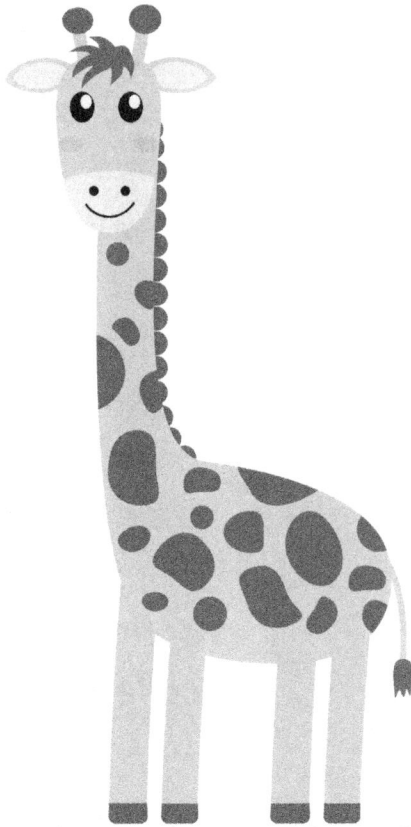

#49 Did you know? Giraffes sleep for around 40 minutes per day!

In captivity Giraffes can sleep for roughly 4.6 hours per day but in the wild they sleep for around 40 minutes, in the form of short naps, just a few minutes at a time! This is so they can stay alert and react quickly to predators when needed! Did you also know that giraffes have dark coloured tongues (black, blue or purple) and it is believed this prevents the tongue from sunburn!

#50 Did you know? Starfish are not actually fish!

As they have no tail, gills, fins or backbone (making them an invertebrate) they are actually echinoderms. There are around 2000 species of starfish. Commonly they have 5 arms, however some starfish can have up to 40 arms! They have no brain and no blood! How strange!

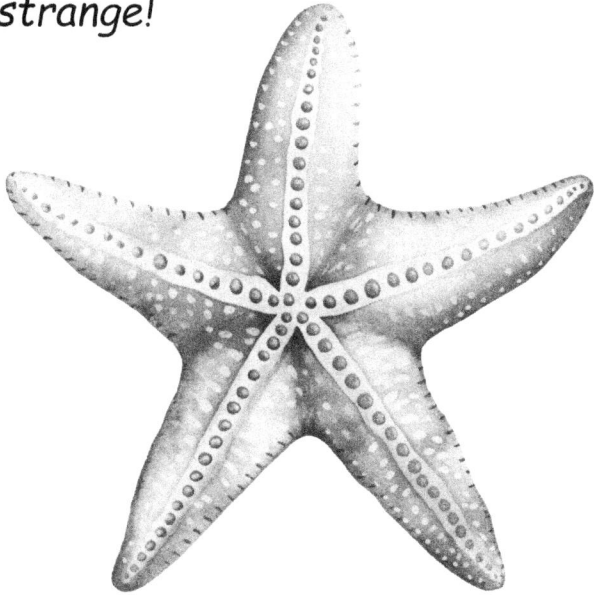

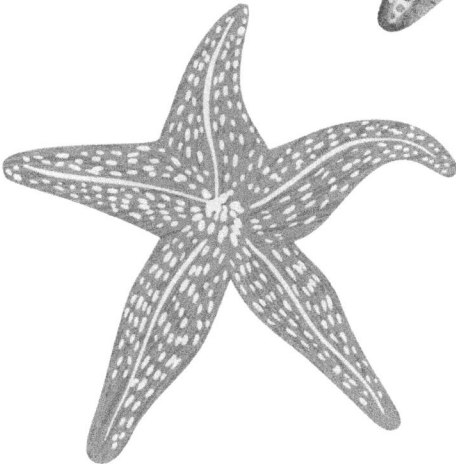

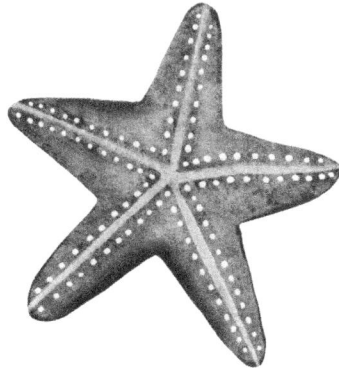

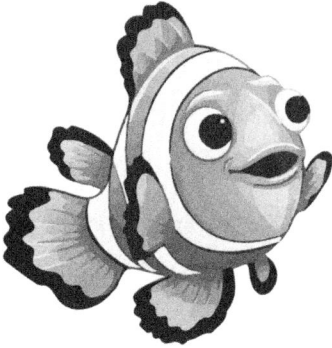

#51 Did you know? All Clownfish are born male! *They all start life as a male but have the ability to change to a female later in life. If the dominant female of the group dies or disappears then a male will develop into the female matriarch!*

#52 Did you know? Chickens are descendants of the dinosaurs, in particular - the T-Rex! *Yes its true, our harmless, feathered friend is the closest living relative of the Tyrannosaurus Rex! Chicken DNA is closer linked to this dinosaur in comparison to reptiles such as the alligator.*

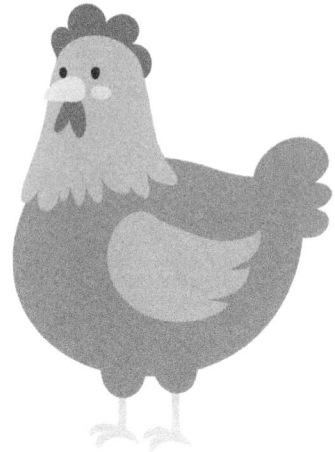

#53 Did you know? Prairie Dogs kiss each other!

These cute rodents are sociable animals who live in tight-knit families. They will greet each other by kissing. A kiss also helps them to identify one another. Pups will kiss their mother for comfort and these funny little animals will only kiss and cuddle their own family members.

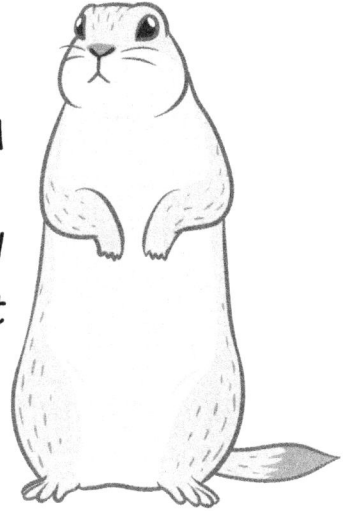

#54 Did you know? A pig cannot look up to the sky!

Due to the structure of their neck and spine, pigs are unable to fully look up at the sky. Pigs only have the ability to tilt their neck, around 45 degrees. They wont mind though, being ground dwellers they are naturally looking down, usually foraging for food!

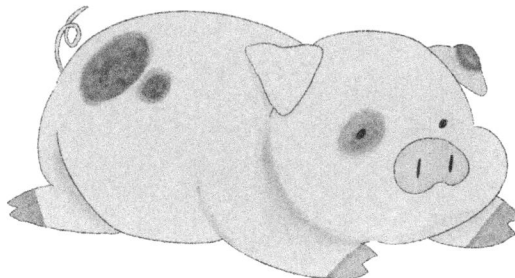

#55 Did you know? A Narwhals unicorn like 'horn' is actually a tooth! *Male narwhals have a long spiralled tooth on the front of their heads. Narwhals only have 2 teeth and 1 of them will then overgrow to become a long 'tusk'. This tusk can grow up to 10 feet in length! Some females can grow a tusk too but not often and on very rare occasions a male can grow 2 tusks!*

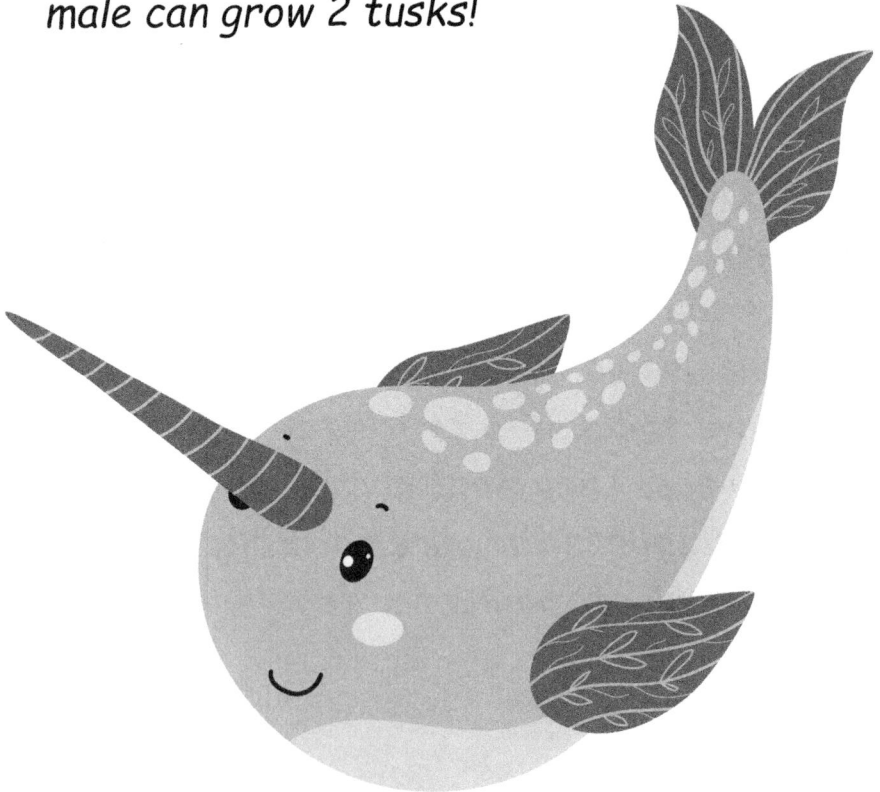

#56 Did you know? A group of Gorillas is called a 'troop'!

Gorillas live in groups, known as troops! These troops are filled with family members. They will always contain a dominant male, several females and their offspring (babies). The male gorilla is called a silverback and he will make all the important decisions for the troop, his role is also to protect the family from any threats. Did you know that male gorillas have up to 10 times the strength of a human! This means they are very capable of tearing down banana trees when needed.

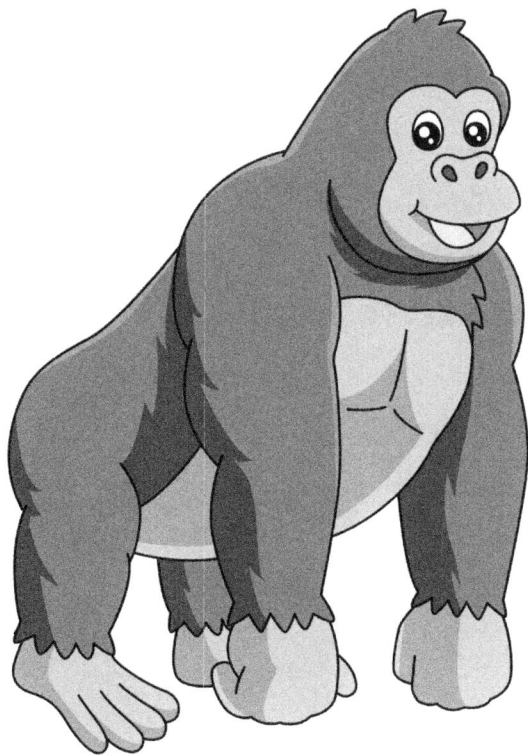

#57 Did you know? Wombat poop is shaped like a cube!

Gross but true! Wombats are the only known species to have cube shaped poop. It is believed that this occurs because wombats mark their territory with their poop, so having a unique cube design prevents it from rolling away!

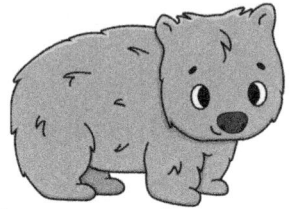

#58 Did you know? Cheetahs are the fastest land animal in the world!

Cheetahs can reach speeds of up to 70 miles per hour (112 kilometres). They can go from 0 to 60 miles per hour in as little as 3 seconds, which is faster than some sports cars, however they can only maintain this amazing speed for around 200-300 metres.

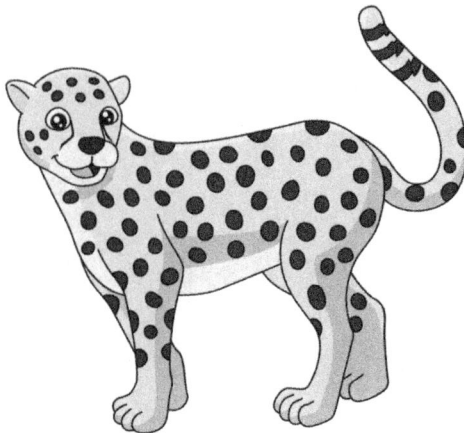

#59 Did you know? Snails can sleep for up to 3 years without waking up!
Snails can hibernate for up to 3 years, they can do this when the climate is too cold and food sources are limited. They will slow their heart rate and their metabolism down so they do not need to eat or move, which allows them to conserve energy during this time.

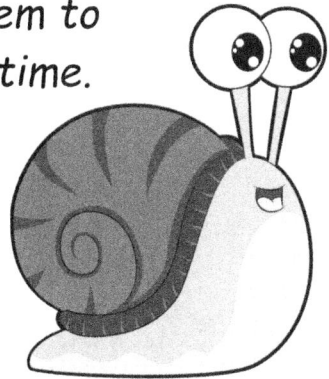

#60 Did you know? Hagfish are the slimiest animal in the world!
Hagfish are strange animals, they live at the bottom of the ocean and have eel-like bodies. They have 4 hearts and no spine or real bones in their body therefore they can literally tie themselves in knots. When they are afraid or threatened by predators, they produce slime as a defence!

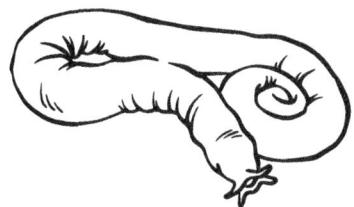

#61 Did you know? a Horned Lizard can shoot blood from its eyes!

They have strong amour to protect themselves from predators but that's not all, if they feel threatened they can also shoot blood from their eyes! Although gross, its pretty cool too as this can fire out, reaching up to 3 feet away!

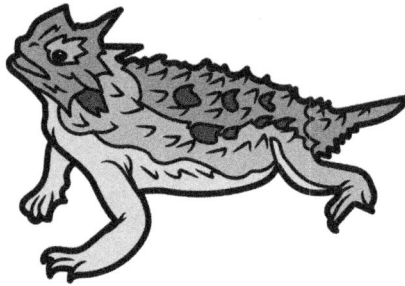

#62 Did you know? Swans will partner for life!

When a male and female swan are together this will be a life long partnership. When they have their babies (cygnets) both mum and dad will take turns watching over them. Swans become very aggressive when guarding their babies, even carrying them on their back to keep them close by!
How cute!

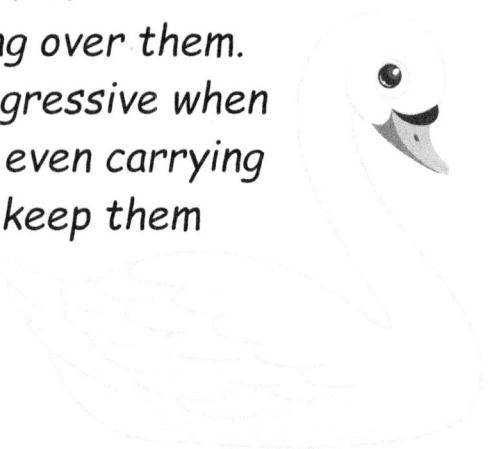

#63 Did you know? A Horse can't breathe through its mouth!

Horses are obligate nasal breathers which means they can only breath through their nostrils, unlike humans who can breathe through both our mouth and nose! This is because the pathway between a horses mouth and lungs is blocked off so they don't accidentally get food into their lungs!

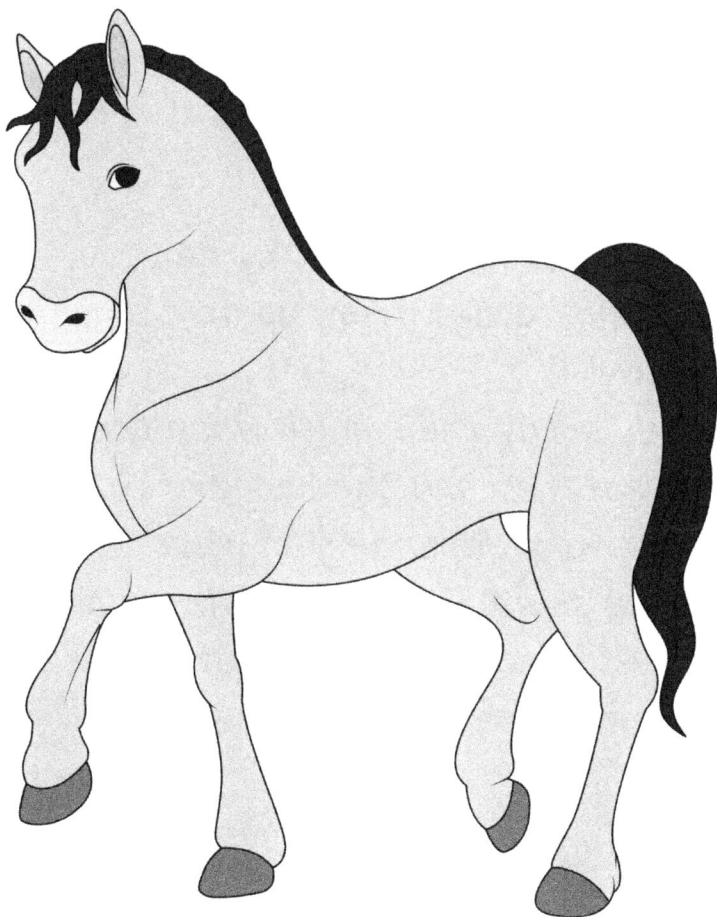

#64 Did you know? Pumas, Cougars and Mountain Lions are all the same species!

This animal actuals holds the record for the mammal with the most names (40 in total) but it also holds the world record for the highest jump (from stand still) at 7 metres (23 feet)!

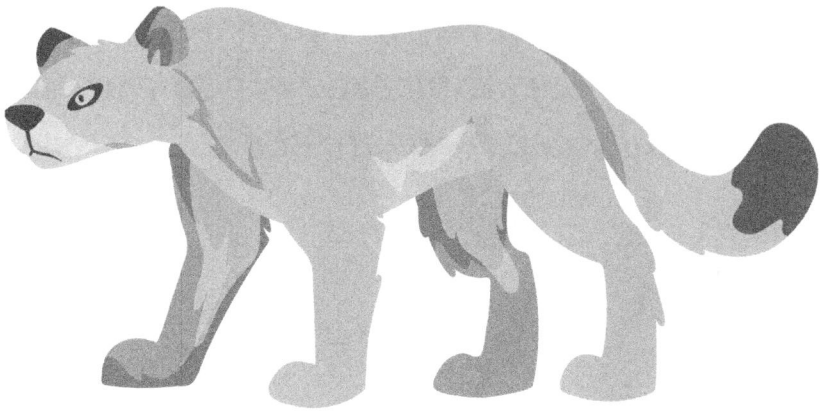

#65 Did you know? Skunks can spray their target from up to 15 feet away!

They only spray their musk when they feel threatened and the range of spray can vary depending on what species of skunk but mostly they can reach 10-15 feet fairly accurately, even more if the wind is in their favour!

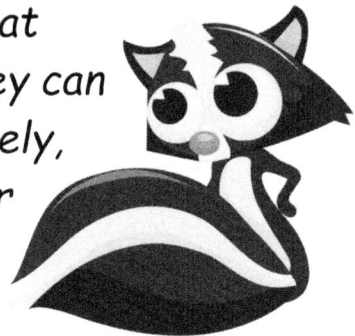

#66 Did you know? Mantis Shrimp have a fast, powerful punch, at a speed of 50mph!

The Mantis shrimp has 2 arm like clubs that they use to attack prey. They have the striking force of a bullet and are able to deliver a punch of over 50mph. This means they are able to smash through a crab shell without a problem. Due to packing a punch they are also able to break glass, so aquariums need to be of suitable strength or material to house these crustaceans!

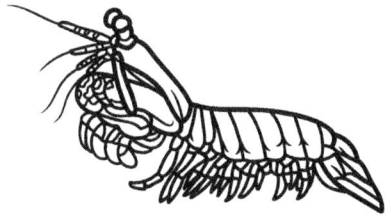

#67 Did you know? Cats cannot taste anything sweet!

Yes, cats are basically sweet blind! Taste buds hold taste receptors and cats do not have the necessary taste receptors that would allow them to taste sweetness! This is because of the lack of gene needed - Tas1r2. Big cats like lions and tigers also cannot taste sweet things!

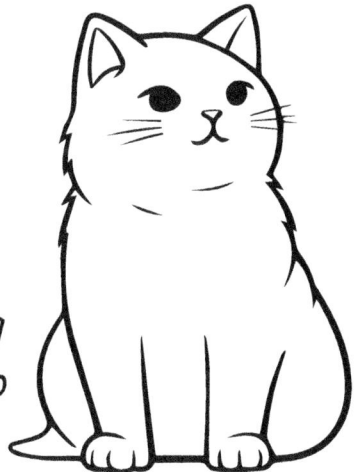

#68 Did you know? Snow Leopards cannot roar!

Unlike large cats like tigers, lions and other wild cats, the snow leopard is not able to roar. They communicate with chuffs, puffs and growls. Thanks to the way their body is designed, with furry padded paws, a thick tail and long strong legs, they can jump as far as 50 feet!

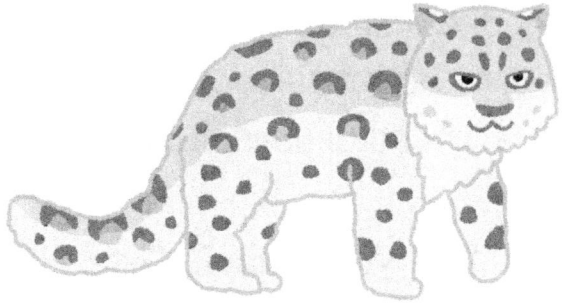

#69 Did you know? A Giant Anteaters tongue can be 2 feet long!

This is the longest tongue of any known mammal! They use this super long tongue to lap up ants and termites and are able to eat 35,000 in just 1 day!! These giant anteaters are also the only know mammal to have no teeth!

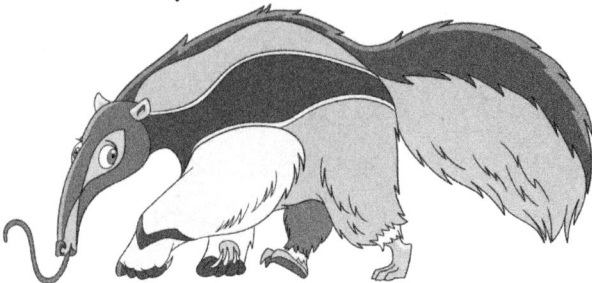

#70 Did you know? Crows can recognise human faces!

Crows are very smart and have great problem solving abilities but what is extra cool is that they can recognise human faces and link them to any positive or negative experiences. They can then communicate this to the other crows within their flock! It is also a fact that crows can hold grudges too!

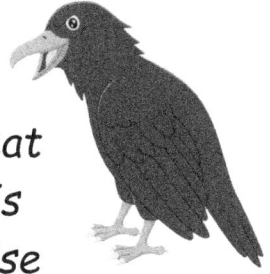

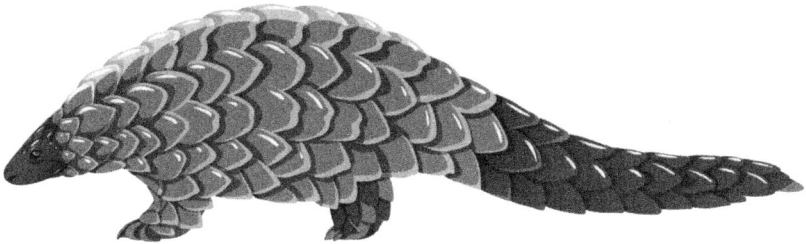

#71 Did you know? Pangolins are the only known scaled mammal!

These unusual animals are referred to as 'scaly anteaters' due to their appearance but are more related to cats and dogs than anteaters! When threatened pangolins roll themselves up into an armoured ball that even lions struggle to bite through. They can also leak a stinky fluid from their glands when defending themselves, similar to a skunk but without the fire power!

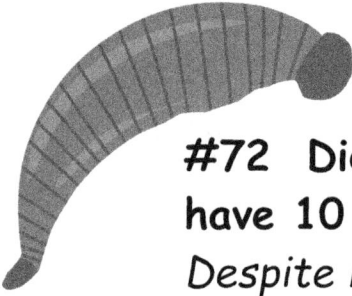

#72 Did you know? Leeches have 10 eyes!
Despite having 10 eyes they have very poor eyesight. They can also range in size and be anywhere between 1cm-30cm!!

#73 Did you know? The Japanese Spider Crab has the largest leg span within the crab world - 12 feet!
This species of marine crab has 8 legs and 2 arms for feeding. Their feeding arms being around 1.5 metres each in length yet their body stops growing at around 15 inches in length. This crabs legs will continue to grow reaching a span of up to 12 feet!

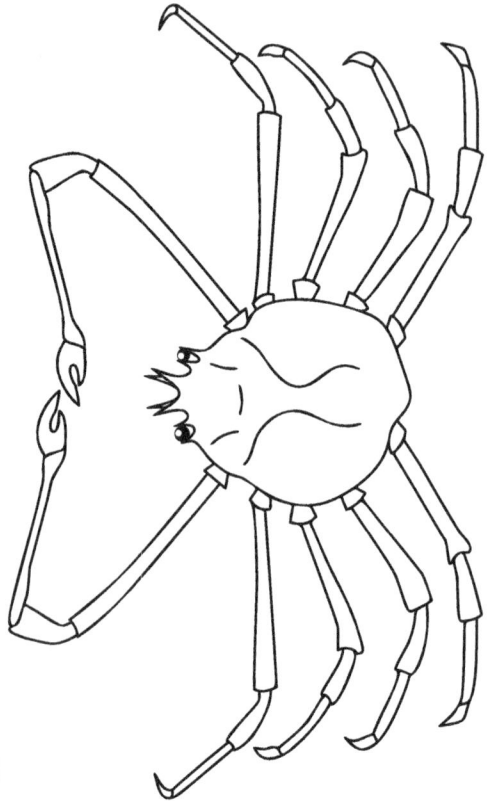

#74 Did you know? Hedgehogs can climb trees!

Yes, when foraging for food these prickly little mammals can climb trees. Hedgehogs can actually swim too! They are also known to be lactose intolerant which means drinking milk can be harmful to them but they are tough... they are actually partially resistance to snake and scorpion venom!

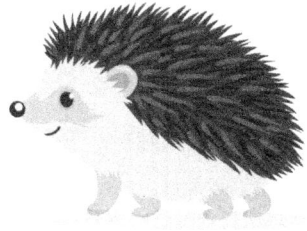

#75 Did you know? Zebra stripes are as unique as finger prints to humans!

Every zebra has their own distinctive striped pattern and despite what some people think they are actually black with white stripes, not white with black stripes! Also, a group of zebra are called a 'dazzle'!

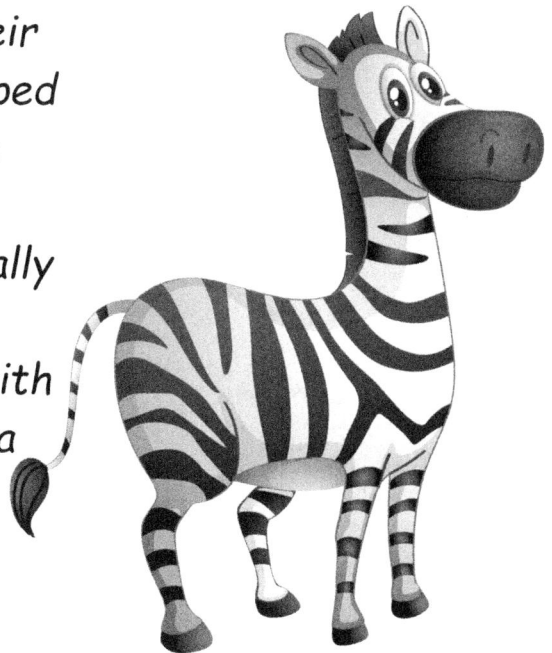

#76 Did you know? Saltwater Crocodiles are the largest of the *crocodile species!*
The biggest saltwater on record (Lolong) was over 20 feet in length! Despite their gigantic body their brains are only the size of a walnut! But don't let the size of their brains fool you as they are one of the more intelligent reptile breeds!

Crocodiles cannot stick out their tongue but have anywhere between 60-100 teeth depending on the species. They are constantly replacing teeth too therefore it is believed crocodiles can have up to 2000 throughout their lifetime!

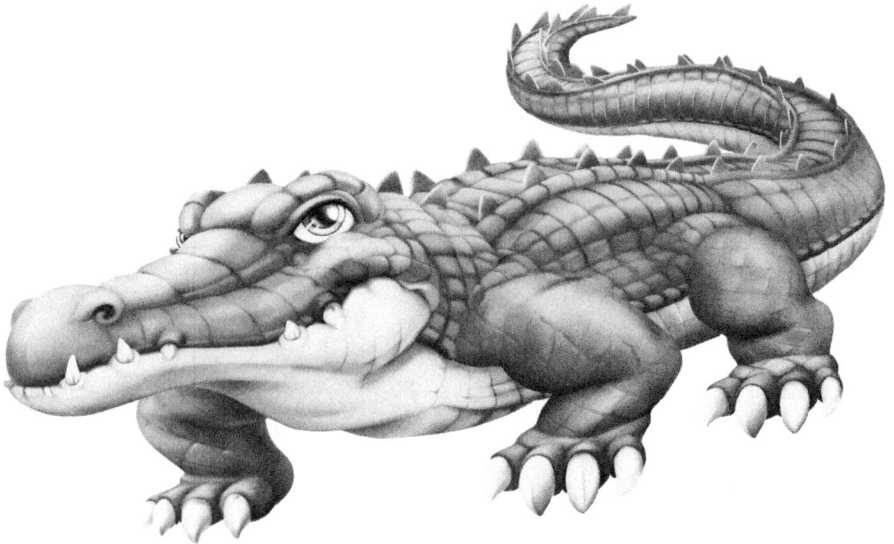

#77 Did you know? Ladybugs cannot fly in cold weather!

Yes these dotty little creatures cannot fly when the temperature is below 55°F (13°C). When they do fly they flap their wings around 85 times per second and can fly up to a speed of 37miles per hour, they can also swim when necessary too!

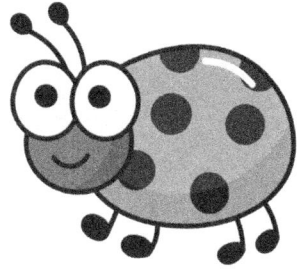

#78 Did you know? Hamsters actually live in the wild!

Not only do these little furry animals live as pets, snuggled up in their cage, but they actually live in the wild throughout various part of the world, including Europe, Asia and the Middle East!

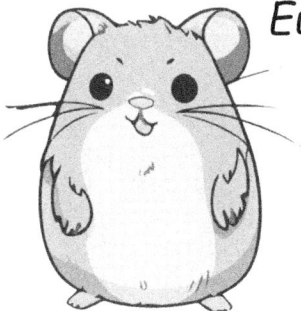

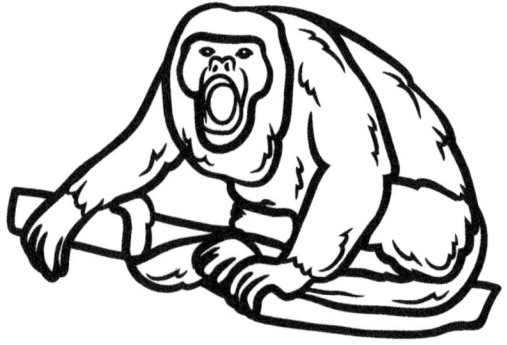

#79 Did you know? Howler Monkeys can be heard from 3 miles away!

Due to their howl like sound they are named 'howler' monkeys, but their calls are so loud they can be heard up to 3 miles away! They have prehensile tails which means their tails can grip, so they can use them as a fifth limb. How handy!

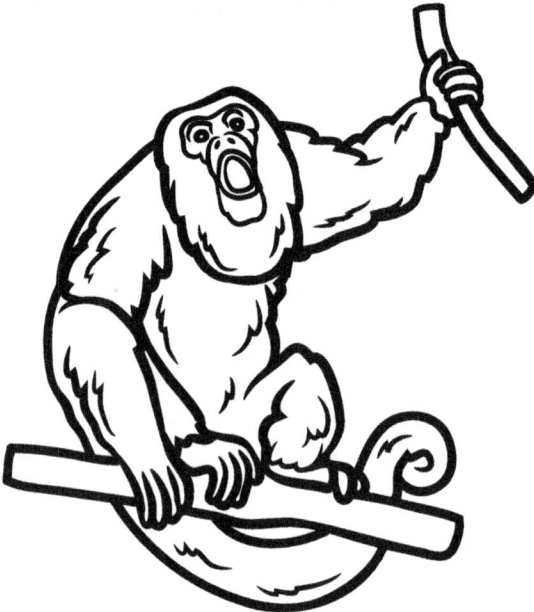

#80 Did you know? Wolf pups are born with blue eyes!

All wolf pups, even artic wolf pups are born with blue eyes. After a few weeks when they begin to develop and grow, their eyes will then change to their adult colour!

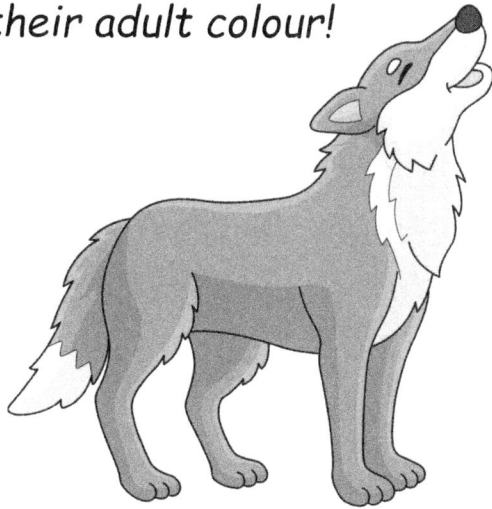

#81 Did you know? A Dung Beetle can roll and pull a gigantic 1141 times its own body weight!

Yep, as gross at these insects are, rolling up and eating dung (poo) from other animals, they are incredibly strong! This strength is the equivalent of a person pulling 6 double decker buses!!

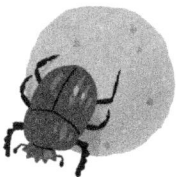

#82 Did you know? The smallest fox in the world is the Fennic Fox?

Also known as the desert fox, due to living in a desert environment. Being small they weigh between just 2.2-3.3 pounds. They have thick fur that protects them in the harsh desert conditions and they have very large ears that radiate body heat, meaning they release heat to help keep the Fennic fox cool and comfortable!

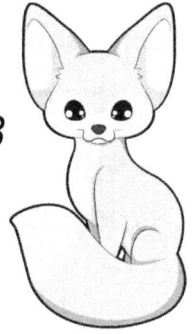

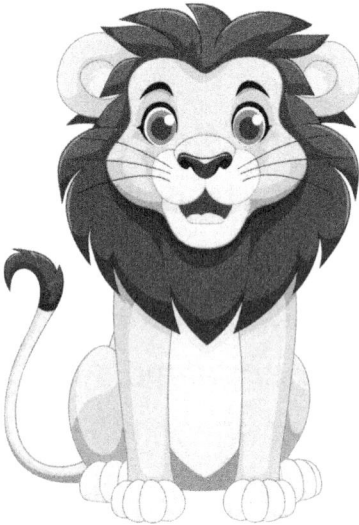

#83 Did you know? An adult lions roar can be heard from up to 5 miles away!

The adult male has the loudest roar and uses this to communicate his power and strength. Did you also know that lions are referred to as the 'king of the jungle'. BUT...Lions do not live in jungles! They live in grassland, savanna and open woodland!

#84 Did you know camels don't have humps when they are born!
Yes they are without humps at birth but at around 10 months they begin to develop their humps. As well as humps, did you know camels have 3 sets of eyelids, 2 rows of eyelashes and the ability to close their nostrils in a sandstorm!

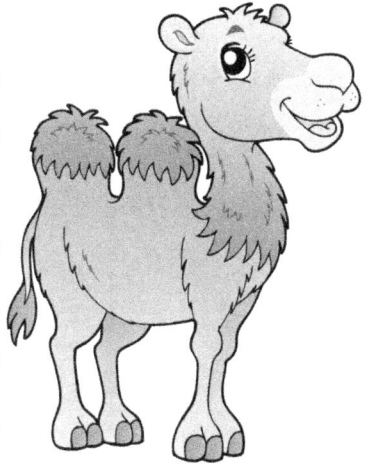

#85 Did you know? The Anaconda is the largest snake in the world! *They can measure between 6-9 metres in length and weigh up to 227kg, that's about 3 times the weight of a kangaroo! Interestingly, the females are much bigger than the males and unlike other snake species that lay eggs, anacondas will instead give birth to live baby snakes!*

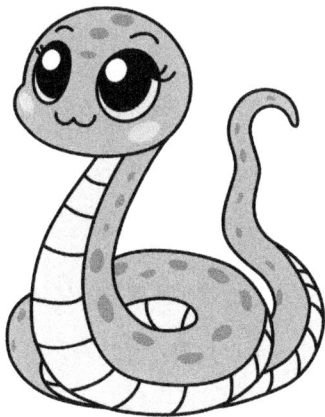

**#86 Did you know?
The largest Rhino is the White Rhino, weighing up to 2500kg which is the equivalent of 30 adults!** *Also, despite there being species named the 'white rhino' and the 'black rhino' they are both grey in colour and both have 2 horns. Even though they are so big, they don't eat any meat, they simply eat plants and grass which means they are herbivores!*

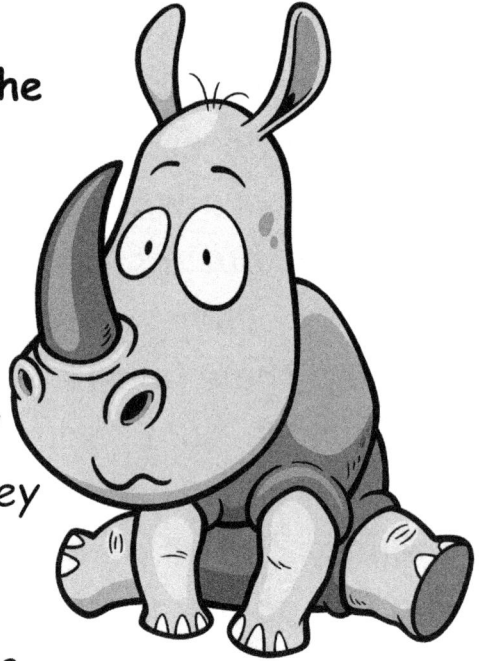

**#87 Did you know?
Beavers teeth are orange!**
This is not because they haven't brushed their teeth properly. It is because their teeth contain iron which makes them extra strong to gnaw through trees!

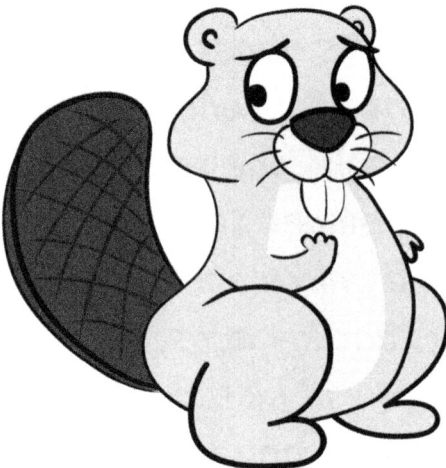

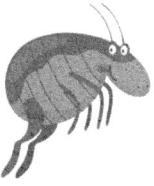

#88 Did you know? A Flea can jump distances 200 times their own body length!

If we could do this as humans, we would be able to jump around 360 metres. That's like jumping the length of 25 buses all lined up together!

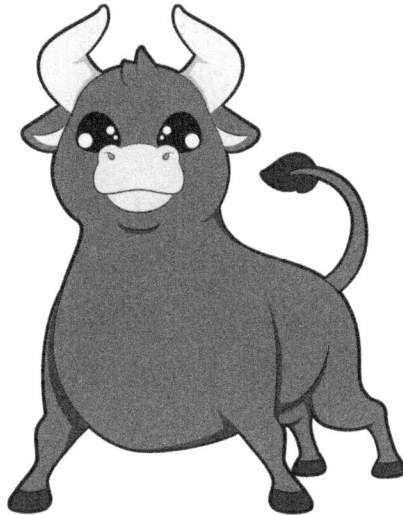

#89 Did you know? That a Bull cannot see the colour red!

Ever heard the phrase 'like a red rag to a bull'? There is a notion that bulls are enraged by the colour red, however bulls are dichromats (meaning they have a type of colour blindness) leaving them unable to actually see the colour red!

#90 Did you know? That a Maned Wolf is not a wolf!

Yes the maned wolf that looks more like a fox, is neither a wolf or a fox! With its long legs, reddish fur and large ears, it is the only species of a unique genus - chrysocyon, meaning 'golden dog' in ancient greek.

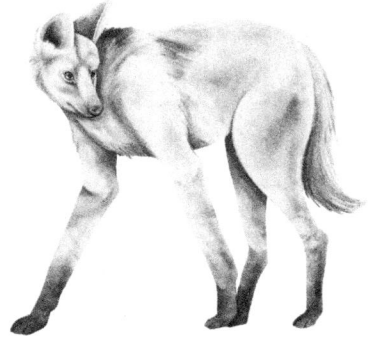

#91 Did you know? The Colossal Squid has the biggest eyes of the entire animal kingdom!

Although it is not the longest squid in the world (it is 2nd to the giant squid) the colossal squid can weigh up to 700kg - the same weight as 4 lions! They reach up to 33feet in length and have eyeballs the size of basketballs! Despite their enormous size, female colossal squid lay very tiny eggs (around 3mm across) but it is believed that they lay up to 4.2 millions eggs!

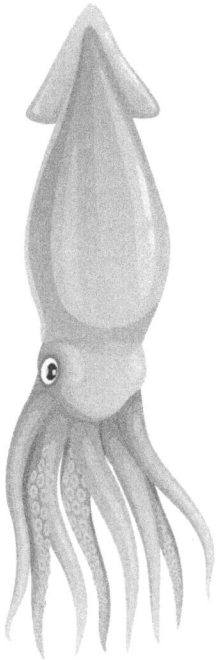

#92 Did you know? The Star-nosed Mole has the most sensitive touch of any mammal!

These weird yet fascinating creatures have 22 rays (little tentacles) on their nose that move around touching its surroundings, acting as tiny sensors. With over 25,000 sensory receptors and each tiny touch having 100,000 nerve fibres sending information to the moles brain, you can see why they have such a sensitive touch! To compare, these nerve fibres are 5 times more than what is in the human hand! Star-nosed moles use these rays to rapidly identify food and hoover it up just as quickly too. This magnificent mole can also swim and has the ability to smell under water. They do this by blowing air bubbles into the water (to collect a scent), then suck the bubbles back up into their nose!

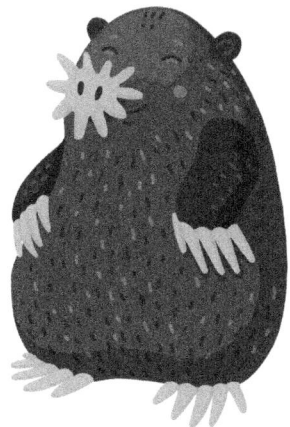

#93 Did you know? The Kiwi is the only bird in the world with nostrils on the tip of its beak!
They are the national bird of New Zealand. Kiwis are flightless birds that have whiskers and a long beak with nostrils at the tip, this help them locate food. Kiwis are mostly nocturnal which means they are more active in the night rather than the day. Kiwis do not have good eyesight so rely on their hearing, touch and their great sense of smell!

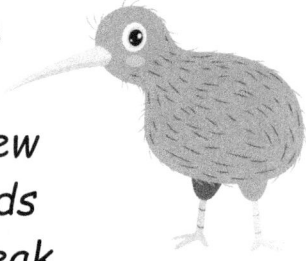

#94 Did you know? That Coral is actually an animal!
Some may think these are colourful plants or rocks, but no, they are actually living sea animals that stay in one place and are home to many other sea creatures like seahorses, clams and turtles!

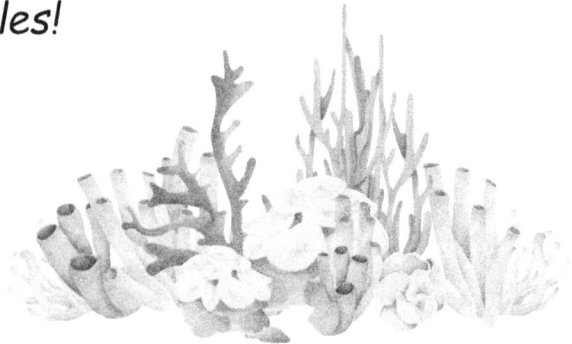

#95 Did you know? Komodo Dragons are lizards, not dragons!

Of course they are not dragons but they do have a split tongue like a dragon would have! Komodo Dragons are the largest lizard in the world, they are fierce, fast and strong! They even have their own built-in armour. They have lots of tiny chain mail bones just under their skin which helps protect them. This is the ultimate lizard, with long claws, sharp teeth and a powerful tail. The tail is as long as their body and their tail alone is strong enough to take down a deer! They can swim and are also venomous- not an animal to be messed with!

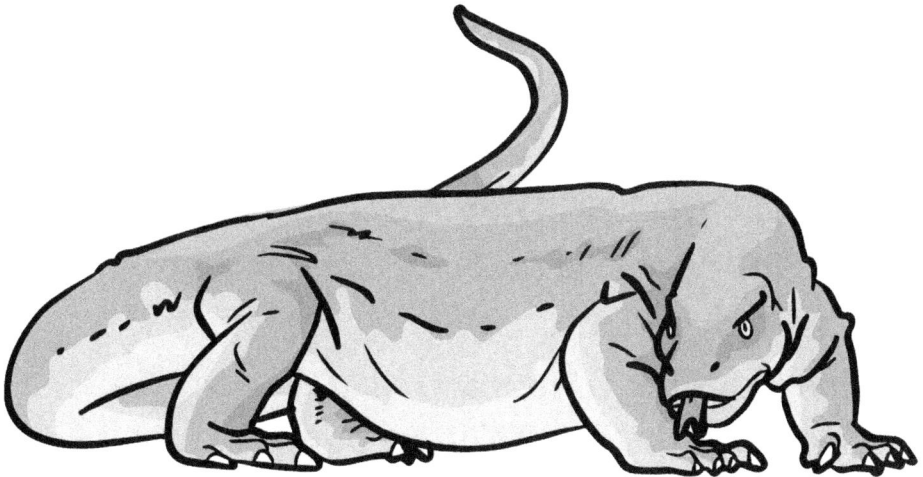

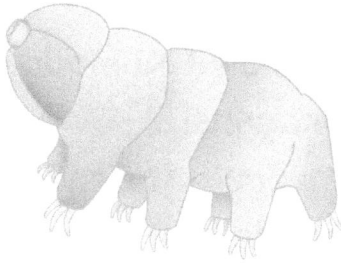

#96 Did you know? Tardigrades are capable of surviving in space!

Tardigrades (sometimes called 'water bears' or 'moss piglets') have been on earth for around 600 million years - this means they are even older than dinosaurs, by about 400 million years! They are only microscopic in size but mighty! Tardigrades can live in conditions that would certainly kill most animals. Despite living in water they can go without it for years! They can survive in extreme dryness, and extreme temperatures. They have survived way below freezing and can even withstand being heated to boiling point. Most impressively, they can also survive the vacuum and radiation of outer space! unbelievable!

#97 Did you know? A Manatee is also referred to as a 'Sea Cow'!

The reason they are known as sea cows is due to their similarities. Both animals have a slow paced life, a large build and a docile nature, and they both like to spend their days grazing (both being herbivores). The Manatee is a gentle giant who lives in warm shallow waters eating seagrass and underwater plants. Its closest living relative is actually an elephant!

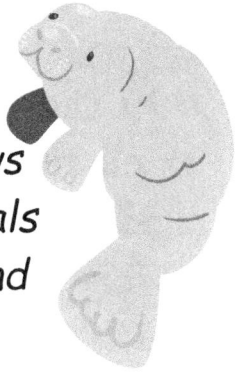

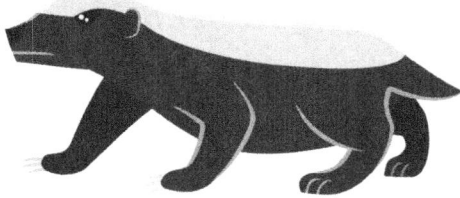

#98 Did you know? Honey Badgers are not actually badgers!

They are part of the weasel family and despite their sweet name, their nature is quite the opposite! Known for its fearlessness and aggressive manner, honey badgers are intelligent, tough creatures, with tough skin, sharp claws and a strong jaw that can crack through a turtles shell! They are named honey badgers as they love to raid honey bee nests, not for the honey itself but the bee larvae found within the honey!

#99 Did you know? Silkworms are not worms at all they are actually caterpillars that produce the amazing fabric, silk!

Before a silkworm turns into a beautiful silk moth, it feeds on large amounts of mulberry leaves, this helps with growth and silk production. It builds its cocoon over 2-3 days using a single continuous thread of raw silk that can measure up to 900 metres long! Once the cocoon is formed, they are harvested for silk production! Fascinating!

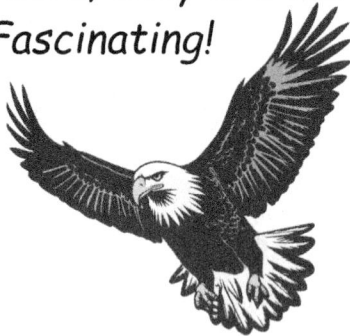

#100 Did you know? An Eagles vision is up to 5 times greater than a humans!

Due to their excellent vision eagles can spot prey up to 2 miles away! As well as impressive sight and speed (reaching up to 100 miles per hour during a dive) they also have an impressive wingspan too. A Bald Eagle (which is not actually bald) can have a wingspan of up to 8 feet! Also did you know baby eagles are called eaglets?!